The Mediterranean Diet

Weight loss for beginners

Alex Junior

Table of Contents

Introduction

The Mediterranean diet has a rich history and a lot of background. It's proven itself to be the best thing you can do for your body, especially if you have some health concerns about where your body is heading!

Rather than being based on pseudoscience, the Mediterranean diet has a rich history, filled with interesting points. As you might imagine from the name, the Mediterranean diet originates from the countries that surround the Mediterranean Sea. This includes Greece, Italy, parts of the middle east, and parts of Africa. The coastal regions of Spain and France also seem to follow this diet.

This is less of a diet and more about the eating pattern created thanks to a culture surrounded by sea. Its use is documented in most ancient civilizations in this area... and there were quite a few of them. Think of Ancient Greece, Rome, the Sumerians, the Babylonians, and more! This being said, one can't really tell when these diets became a reality for people.

While the word diet keeps being used, it isn't an accurate one. The Mediterranean region has grown to eat this way after thousands of years. This is a cultural eating style passed down through generations of healthy eating. The sea itself has given life to this area. There is plenty of fish that can be found in the water. The sea has soaked into the soil, making it rich and able to grow whatever the people need. Finally, the area's ample weather means that they can produce a ton of food! It's not a custom in these areas to get good that has been chemically treated in any way. Most of the people within these regions are actually distrustful of this! It's also not common in these areas to purchase imported food! It's more expensive and there isn't a need for it. Instead, one can simply get their food straight from the farm. It's less expensive to do this, and people are healthier as a result.

From this, you can imagine that a huge part of the Mediterranean diet is fruits and vegetables. Grains and legumes are grown easily and eaten often as well! Herbs and spices are a part of the diet too! Finally, the Mediterranean diet is high in fat content, but not animal fat. Most of their cooking is done with olive oil, a healthier natural fat.

With this diet, it may be a good idea to consider what type of changes you want to make. First, there is the food itself. It's fresh and healthy, and it's going to fuel your body–but now you do need to think about how you are going to incorporate this! It's best to not just change a few ingredients of the meals you are having now in order for them to fit into the diet plan. Keep in mind that this is a cultural eating pattern so many meals have already been created to go along with this. Check out some of these meals for yourself. You are going to find a lot of mixed bowls, salads, and other great recipes.

Your lifestyle also matters here. In these regions, a lot of emphases is placed on exercise. In Spain, for example, it's more common to bike and many don't drive unless they have to. There are several other regions out there that make a habit out of regular outdoor exercise time, and it's proven to be very beneficial for them!

Finally, a lot of family time and togetherness is incorporated into these cultures. Family meals are a must when possible, and eating alone almost never happens, even if the meals are just shared with friends.

This is a stark difference when these behaviors are compared to other cultures. Think about your daily life. Do you drive to where you need to be? Is there a way to bike? How often do you get exercise otherwise? In America, that number is stagnant for many people. Changes in habits like these can make a great difference in how the story of your health goes.

Such a change may sound terrifying at first, but I can promise you that it's absolutely worth it, and once you get into the swing of the new diet, it's easy. The exercise may be harder to work into your day at first, but with time it will get easier. It will become easier to do the exercises as your body gets healthier. As your body's health increases, you will also find that you can do more with your exercises. This might mean that when you are jogging, you can go a further distance in roughly the same amount of time or that as you lift weights, you find that the weight you lift gets heavier. If you are able to ride your bike to work thanks to it being a short distance away, then each time you do so, you are likely to notice that the time it will take you to do this gets shorter and shorter with each trip.

These changes don't just apply to exercise. It will get easier and more comfortable to have and spend that time with your family. If your family doesn't do this right now, then it might be awkward at first. But, once you get into the habit of doing these things, it will become comfortable for you. Additionally, it's likely to become an enjoyable time for your family.

Finally, the food itself is going to have benefits to it! Mediterranean recipes might feel weird at first as you get used to them! Overall though, these dishes tend to be easier to make, and they take less time. If you are worried about the time spent on exercising and other things, this diet may add that time right back through its food preparation.

It's not really possible to tell the future, but we can make an educated guess on what might happen with our health based on how our health has treated us so far, and with what lurks in our family medical history. The Mediterranean diet can help avoid a lot of these things.

One of the major things to note about the Mediterranean diet is also the effect it has on our weight. This diet wasn't designed for weight loss, but that seems to be one of the major perks of following it. This diet stood out to researchers because while parts of the world were suffering from major weight-related issues, this area wasn't.

After trying several different things to improve my health, finding this diet has been my dream! I absolutely love what it's done for me, my health, and my body! Starting with the foods to be consumed, let me introduce you to this diet!

Chapter 1: An Ideal Diet

A huge part of any diet and lifestyle change is–food. Food can be a huge part of a person's health. As we talked about in the previous chapter, there are several things that make the Mediterranean diet unique.

First, the area's structure has been what made this way of eating and living possible in this culture for such a long time. The sea has made the land around them so fertile that vegetable growth is easy and can be done with little to no chemical treatment. The climate can help with this too! It makes it possible to grow enough to sustain the population. Imported foods aren't as trusted in these areas.

This alone plays a major role in a person's health. It's unknown what role the chemicals and GMOs play when it comes to our worsening health, but many are sure that there is a link of some kind there. Imported and packaged foods are even worse, as they will have gone through even more processing.

If you are able to get organic foods, they will be the least processed and have the least amount of chemicals in them. If you're worried about fruits or vegetables going bad, remember that they can be frozen! Some stores sell frozen, organic items as well.

Now, let's be honest! Organic isn't cheap. If your budget doesn't allow for organic items, then that's okay! This way of eating can still be incredibly beneficial to someone who needs a healthy, steady diet. Shop locally if you can and if you're prioritizing, get organic vegetables first. They won't go bad as quickly as fruit will and organic meat are incredibly pricey (and you'll likely be eating less of it anyway)!

Now that we've talked about what to look for in your food, let's talk about what food to look for!

Daily Foods

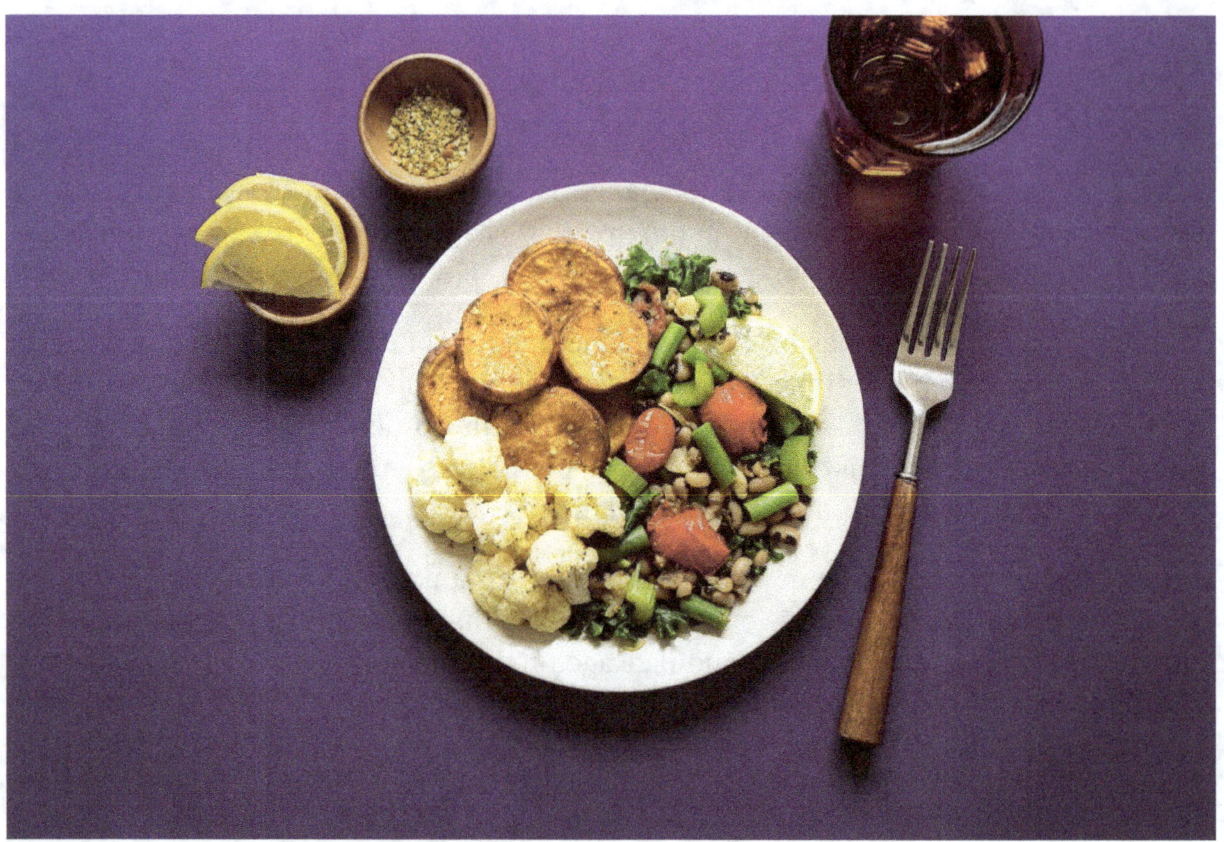

When you look up the Mediterranean diet, you will come across a food pyramid. These are great for setting up your goals and your meals. We are first going to cover the bottom of this pyramid. These are foods that you can and should eat every day!

Vegetables

As you can imagine, vegetables are the first thing on the list. Not only is eating vegetables everyday recommended with this diet, but if you can, you should try to consume them with every meal. In America, we are often called out for having meat be the main part of our food dishes, with vegetables at the side. Experts have recommended the opposite eating pattern for years. Vegetables and other groups should be the main part of the dish, with meat and sides making for some great toppings! Some vegetables to add into your foods include carrots, onions, broccoli, spinach, kale, garlic, zucchini, mushrooms, and of course so many more! Don't forget that frozen vegetables, like peas and frozen broccoli chunks, are also just as great for you, and they can often be found organic as well!

Now, slightly removed from the vegetable family are potatoes, white potatoes, sweet potatoes, yams, and other starchy foods are a part of the Mediterranean diet. They provide a great place for you to get your carbs in, and a small amount of them can be very filling!

Fruits

Fruits are another major part of your everyday diet! Try to have at least three servings a day of fruit, whether that's in the form of a snack, part of the meal, or for dessert. The freshest fruits can satisfy cravings for candy and sweets. Some great fruits to have in your diet include apples, bananas, oranges, grapes, melons, peaches, pears, strawberries, blueberries, and of course, many more!

Whole Grains

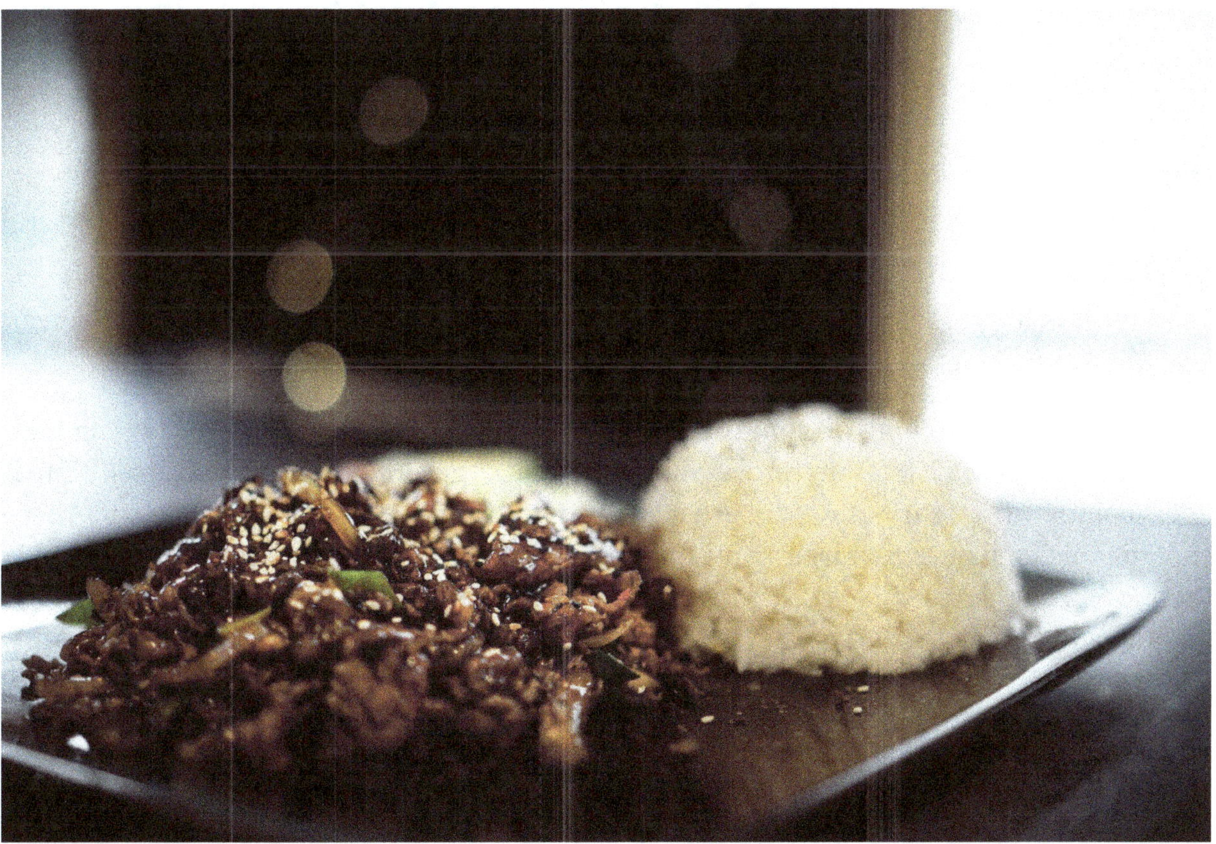

It's now time to distinguish what's a whole grain—and what isn't! Whole grains themselves are hard to make into products, so the white grain was invented. Many products were stripped of their outer shell and other parts in order to get the white part of the grain that they could easily make into something. The trouble is that those shells contained vitamins and minerals that are essential to our health and well-being. Grains are found in bread, pasta, rice, oats, and quinoa. When you are shopping for these products, try to avoid any of the regular items. Instead, look for things like whole grain or whole wheat bread, whole wheat pasta, brown rice, or whole oats. Most quinoa grains aren't stripped to this level so it's often okay to consume this in any form!

Legumes

Have you heard the term legumes before? Those who haven't done food research in the past may be unfamiliar with this term and that's okay! Legumes essentially refer to beans. Well—non-processed beans. Baked beans, for example, are not considered legumes due to their processing and high sugar contents. Legumes consist of lentils, chickpeas, black beans, kidney beans, lima beans, white beans, black-eyed peas (yes, that's a real bean), and many more! Beans provide a great source of protein for your diet, which is especially important since this asks you to reconsider how much meat you take in!

Healthy Fats

Healthy fats are a major part of the Mediterranean diet! It's not really Mediterranean without there being some cooking oil involved in the process of making it.

It's thanks to the cooking oil that the Mediterranean diet can get away with being high fat. Most of it hasn't had any processing beyond the production of the oil itself, but it does come with great taste and great benefits! Examples of healthy fats and these cooking oils include extra virgin olive oil, olives, avocados, and avocado oil. Canola oil is their opposing force. It's more processed with more chemicals added, so it's a less healthy alternative.

Herbs and Spices

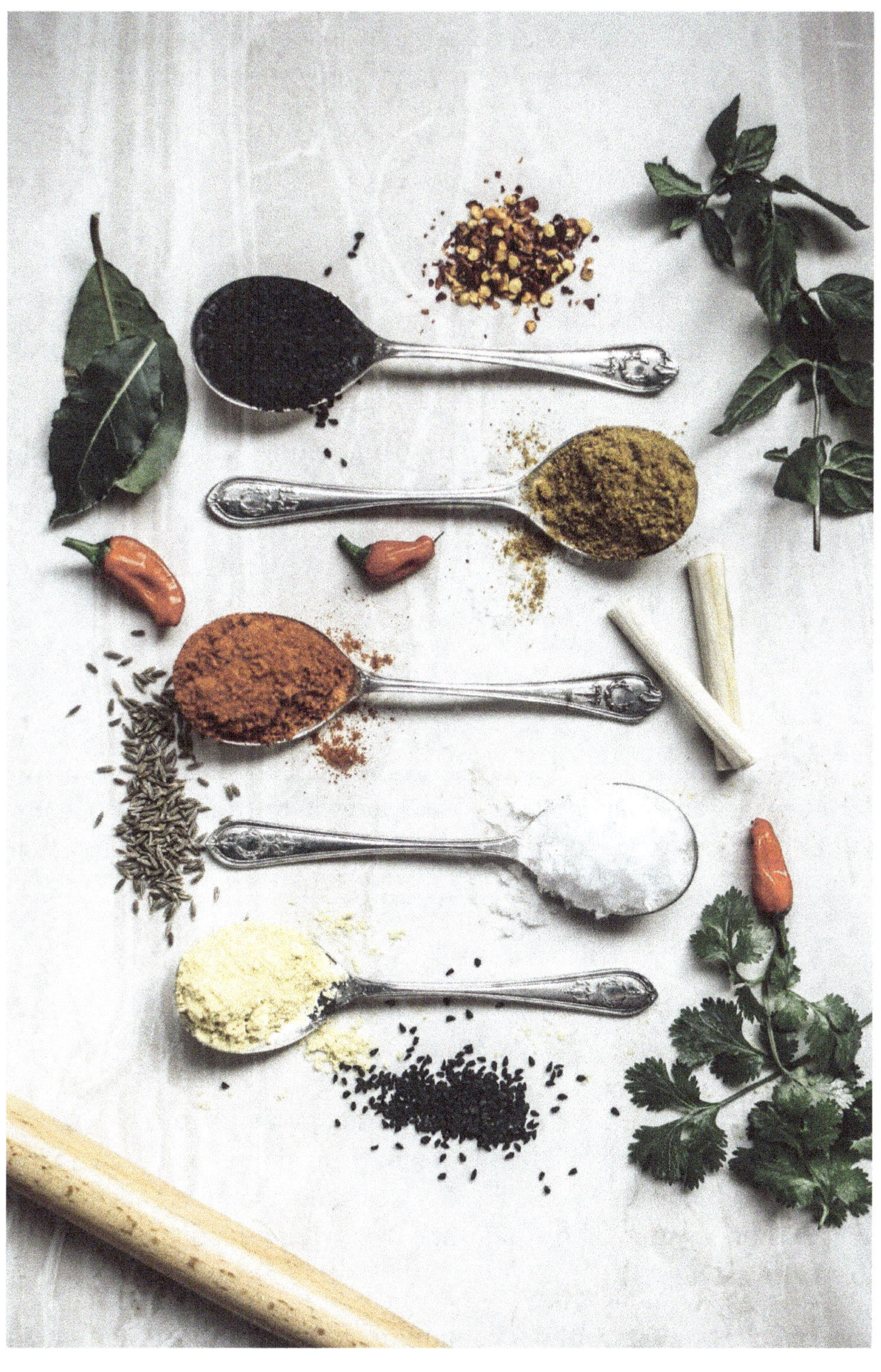

The final thing that stands at the bottom of the food pyramid is herbs... and spices. Add these to every dish. I know that you have a cabinet full of unused spices, so let's make use of them.

Don't forget your herbs either. Herbs can be found fresh in just about every supermarket out there. If you don't like that, it's very easy to grow an herb garden with just a few spare boxes!

Zero and Low-Calorie Beverages

Let me start out by saying that you do not need to consume these multiple times a day as a part of the diet, but if you want to, you can! These will not harm the diet.

These beverages include coffee and tea, which many of us enjoy. They also include water, low-calorie juice, and wine (in smaller quantities).

Three Times a Week

This next food group is also going to be a major part of the Mediterranean diet–it will just be enjoyed less often! You can consume these foods anywhere from daily to about three times a week. With daily consumption, they might be a part of one meal on that day!

Fish and Shellfish

Our first group is fish and shellfish. There are already so many fruits and vegetables wherever they need to go, but when someone in the Mediterranean region has a craving for meat, fish is readily available. The Mediterranean sea is enormous, and there is plenty of salmon, tuna, shrimp, oysters, and whatever other type of food you can think of. It's readily available in this area!

Fish happens to be rich in Omega-3 fats without containing much (if any) of the fat that tends to harm our bodies. Because of this, it's a great source of protein for us as well as a source of vitamins and minerals.

Some great seafood options include salmon, sardines, mackerel, trout, tuna, cod, shrimp, oysters, mussels, and clam!

Seeds

Seeds are another thing! Seeds can provide vitamins and minerals for you. They can either be snacks that you eat during the day, something you add to a salad to give it crunch, something you add to a smoothie to give it a balanced kick, or in the case of pumpkin seeds, you can bake them for a dessert. Chia and hemp seeds can also be made into cereals and other breakfast dishes. Some common seeds include sunflower seeds, pumpkin seeds, chia seeds, and hemp seeds.

Nuts

Finally, on this list is nuts. Nuts and nut butter like peanut butter or almond butter can be high in their nutritional value, as well as containing the vitamins and minerals that we all need to sustain our bodies! Some good nuts to keep in mind are almonds, walnuts, cashews, pistachios, macadamia nuts, and peanuts. If you can, try to look for more pure, less processed nut types.

Two Times a Week

Our next group of foods is still found in the Mediterranean region, but not as much. With the wealth of other foods, it was never consumed as often. Today, these foods are not considered bad for you, but many try to suggest healthier alternatives instead.

Poultry

Poultry refers to your white meats, mainly including turkey and chicken (other birds are included in this too but they are rarely sold). These meats start having some negative effects on our cholesterol and blood pressure if we consume them in excess. The reason this happens is that these meats contain more of the omega-6 fat that fish doesn't have and less of the beneficial omega-3 fat.

Bird meat isn't as easy to get a hold of in these areas compared to fish, shellfish, and fruits and vegetables, and the average family wouldn't have had access to it until agriculture and larger production became mainstream.

It is still enjoyed in about three meals a week for the average family.

Eggs

Now, in America, eggs are a part of an everyday breakfast, and for good reason. They do contain a good amount of protein in return for a lower calorie count. Unfortunately, they also contain a lot in the way of omega-6 fats (while still not holding much in the way of omega-3s). Because of this, many dieticians who follow this diet recommend other breakfasts instead. Eggs are best eaten no more than three times a week and if you want to break the habit of having them regularly in the morning, try adding them to a breakfast bowl as an ingredient instead!

Dairy

Finally, we have our dairy products on this list. This includes milk, cheese, yogurt, and anything else made from cow's (or goat) milk. Much like poultry, and for that matter eggs, dairy isn't as easy to come by as some of the other foods available in this region. While dairy does have some of the "need to avoid" omega-6 fats, it also has plenty of vitamins and minerals. Notably, it is a key source of vitamin D. While the Mediterranean culture spends more time outside, and therefore gets more natural vitamin D, this isn't true in a lot of cultures. If you work a job that keeps you indoors, try having some supplements, or upping your dairy intake to three to four times a week.

If you are able to work outdoors though, it's good to cut back on dairy items.

Once a Week

These next items are best consumed once a week or less. For various reasons, the Mediterranean diet has not featured these foods very much. This has happened naturally due to the area, with the people's health having little to do influence this. Well, the result is that they seem to be doing better with their health than most parts of the world are.

Red Meats

In this region of the world, red meat has never been a major part of the diet. Records show that only the rich were the only ones who really had any access to red meat, and even then, they didn't have it or need it very often. There were so many other options that were in more abundance that could just as easily be created into a delicacy.

Today, red meat has been linked to a host of heart issues and issues with organ function within the body. It's very high in omega-6 fat. As a part of the diet, it is consumed once a week at most. Red meat includes any kind of beef, lamb, pork, veal, and most other animal meats (with the exception of bird meats).

Sweets

Finally, we get to talk about sweets. You don't have to eliminate sweets in your diet. They are still consumed in the Mediterranean region. This is especially true for pastries, which are often a featured breakfast item in Italy.

Sweets, as we know them in most parts of the world, are overloaded with sugar and heavily processed items. The candy by the checkout lane or the twinkies in the desert section is much different than an Italian pastry. Sweets like these are eaten once a week, or often less.

If you find yourself with a sweet tooth, you can try some fresh fruit. Organic fruit can often be sweeter. If you are craving sugar specifically, stop by a local bakery with fresh pastries once or twice a week. These will be better for you in the long run!

Snacks for the Mediterranean Diet

Let's be real! Many people get hungry in the middle of the day. In the past, when I've faced this afternoon hunger, the snacks I reached for weren't at all healthy. While, at the time, I didn't think it to be a big deal, I've been proven wrong. They hurt your health and destroy your energy levels. Below are some better options that I have discovered that fit in well with the Mediterranean diet.

Nuts. A small amount of nuts (half a cup) can be filling, provide protein, and give you energy!

Fruit. A small amount of fruit (half an apple, some peach slices, a slice of cantaloupe, or half a cup to one cup of grapes) can be another great snack. This puts more fruit in your diet, and the energy you get from it will last longer. Don't forget that berries of all kinds are a part of this group too.

Hummus and veggies. Carrots, celery, and peppers are often dipped in hummus, which you can buy or easily make with chickpeas. This creates another great snack for you to have! It also has protein!

Greek Yogurt can be a great snack. A cup of yogurt can have a lot of benefits and it will restore your hunger and energy levels.

Hard-boiled egg. This is a great source of protein that you can add some spice too if you don't like them plain!

Almond butter. Almond butter is yet another great source of protein. It can be applied on whole wheat toast, or eaten with fruits or vegetables!

Guacamole and vegetables. Made from avocados, guacamole can be a great source of healthy fat for your diet. Again, you can have it with vegetables, or if you are looking for a breakfast idea, try it on whole wheat toast!

Cottage cheese and fruit. You can mix it up or keep it separate, but this is another delicious way of creating a satisfying snack for yourself!

Chia Pudding. Our last friend here is for those looking to satisfy their sweet tooth without resorting to sweets. This can be really good!

Now that I've gone over the major food groups and where they fall on this diet pyramid, it's time to talk about what specific foods hold up the Mediterranean diet!

Chapter 2: Foods to Rely On

Let's talk a little bit about why this diet has gained so much popularity.

Face it, most of the world is seeing a crisis in obesity, heart disease, and other issues that have been linked to food. While heart disease is a number one killer in some countries, the Mediterranean region sees very little of it! This drew the world's attention to their diet. While they eat the same foods we do, they eat them differently. Because of this, they've avoided many of these problems. Through research, some foods in their diet have been determined to bring some benefits with them.

This next list consists of foods that are eaten regularly in the Mediterranean region, but not so much elsewhere in the world. It's these foods, especially, that seem to bring the benefits with them.

Olive Oil

One such food is olive oil. Olive oil is a kind of fat, there is no denying it. Mediterranean cooking involves a ton of olive oil. It's used in cooking meat and sauteing vegetables. It's used in sauces, dips, dressings, and vinaigrette and it's often even used in baking.

Now, an excess of fat in the diet has been found to contribute to things like diabetes, heart disease, and obesity, but the Mediterranean region doesn't have that.

This is found to be because olive oil replaces canola oil, butter, vegetable oil, and more! These are all saturated fats. In other words, the fat has been so processed for ease of use that it's become bad for us. Olive oil is unsaturated fat that doesn't harm us nearly as much.

Tomatoes

Tomatoes are a wonderful thing to have. Whether you see them as a fruit or a vegetable, they can be added to a lot of things. It should be added as often as you can get it in there it seems! Tomatoes produce lycopene, a cancer-reducing mineral. Lycopene has been linked to decreased rates of breast and prostate cancer.

Tomatoes can be added to sandwiches and salads! They can also be added to pasta in a variety of ways! Make your own sauce or add them to a premade sauce! You can add sundried tomatoes to pasta as well!

Salmon

It's thanks to the unique geography of this region that fresh salmon is readily available. For a long time, salmon and other fish have been consumed with almost no thought as to how they might benefit a person and their body. Oh boy, are there benefits though! Salmon has proven to be high in Omega-3 fatty acids. This differs from Omega-6 in that it contains needed vitamins and minerals, and it's easy for your body to process.

Omega-6, on the other hand, is very hard for your body to process. It's often the case that something goes wrong along the way, and as a result, the fat is now somewhere it shouldn't be.

Salmon is one of the main animal products, so this has largely been avoided in the Mediterranean area!

Walnuts

Next on the list is Walnuts! Walnuts contain certain fats that are actually good for your overall heart health (as hard as that might be to imagine). They also contain some powerful minerals. These will balance the bacteria in your gut and lower your overall cholesterol levels!

Chickpeas

Chickpeas can be added to soups, salads, hummus, and more! They carry several minerals we need, including iron, zinc, folate, and magnesium. Additionally, they also contain fiber which is great for your digestive health. It may help with weight loss too!

Arugula

Arugula is great to add to salads, pasta dishes, eggs, and pretty much anything else that you can think of. Arugula is important to get into your diet somewhere, especially if you have diabetes (which is linked to Alzheimer's), or if you have a family history of diabetes or Alzheimers. Arugula has been shown to reduce the risk of you developing this condition.

Pomegranate

This special little fruit is certainly unique from other fruits in the way it's shaped. You can add it as a topping to a lot of things, you can make it into a juice, and you can eat them as a snack! However you chose to enjoy pomegranate is up to you, but you should! It's been shown to have antioxidant powers, meaning that it can prevent some cell damage. It also has anti-inflammatory properties, which allow it to slow and stop swelling within the body. Because of these properties, it's believed to potentially be effective against cancer development.

Lentils

One of the problems of many modern diets is that with all of the added sugar and other things done to process food, it can have a negative effect on our blood sugar levels which can eventually lead to type 2 diabetes. Lentils can be added to soups and salads, and they have been shown to actually lower blood glucose levels within the body.

Farro

Let's start off by telling you what exactly Farro is! Farro is a grain that can be added to or the main part of a variety of dishes.

First of all, there's both fiber and protein in this grain, meeting some essential nutrient requirements for you already! Furthermore, it reduces your risk of picking up several diet-related diseases including, diabetes, heart disease, stroke, and rectal cancer.

Greek Yogurt

Generally, you are eating less dairy with this diet, and that's a beneficial thing. The joy about greek yogurt though is that it offsets some of the worries that regular dairy comes with. For example, dairy is normally higher in saturated fats, but greek yogurt usually isn't. It's lower in all forms of fat because of the way it's been made.

If you are someone who is inside for most of the day, then greek yogurt can be your friend in giving you some needed vitamin D and calcium.

Oats

If eggs are a go-to for breakfast, and you are thinking of trying something else, then it might be worth it to give oats a good go! Oats still have protein in them. They also contain healthy fats for you, and they have iron and various B vitamins. You can make oatmeal, top different breakfast bowls with oats, or do overnight oats (this last one is great if you have early mornings).

Extra Virgin Olive Oil

Yes, this one gets a special place away from the rest of the olive oil family!

If you have a choice between buying regular olive oil and buying extra virgin olive oil, you should aim for the latter. Regular olive oil has been through more processing and may even be mixed with canola or vegetable oil. In addition to containing the benefits that regular olive oil will have, extra virgin olive oil contains oleic acid and a ton of antioxidants, which can reduce inflammation and cancer within your body.

Green, Leafy Vegetables

These include both iceberg and romaine lettuce as well as spinach, kale, and other leafy veggies. As a general rule of thumb, the darker the leaf, the better it is for you!

They contain more vitamins than you would believe. These include vitamin A, Vitamin C, folate, Vitamin K, Iron, calcium, phosphate, and potassium.

These are all essential for our function, and we can get them all in one place!

Berries

Finally, we have to mention berries! Why? First of all, if you are worried about sugar content, then berries should be your way to go. They are not as high in natural sugars as other fruits are. Berries themselves have vitamins and minerals that we need. They tend to help lower blood pressure, and they help keep blood from becoming too thick and creating a clot.

The specific benefits that foods can have are amazing to even me! Now that you have an overview of how to balance the foods you have within this diet and what foods to focus on having, we are going to talk about meal plans. As I mentioned before, the meals for this diet are going to be different from what you are used to. But, don't worry! We are here to help with that!

Chapter 3: A Mediterranean Diet Meal Plan

The Mediterranean diet isn't really like other diets you might have tried in the past. Unlike introducing a diet that someone who is likely from the same culture created, we are introducing an entirely new cultural eating pattern to you, and it's okay if that's going to take a minute to adjust to! To help you out, we have a sample meal plan below!

This meal plan balances through the Mediterranean food pyramid recommendations and it suggests additions for the key items in the diet. It can help you get an idea of what an everyday diet here would look like! All of these are in one portion, but you can easily multiply to get what you need!

Day 1

Start this plan on any day of the week you wish!

Breakfast

Here are some ingredients you will need!

- an egg
- tomatoes
- a slice of whole wheat toast

Now, you have a few options for how you might choose to put these ingredients together!

First, you can either scramble or fry the egg depending on your personal preference. You can also consider cutting a hole in the middle of your bread and putting the egg in there. Next, for the tomatoes, you can simply slice and eat them, or choose to grill them or cook them in a pan. You can layer these ingredients in any way you choose. For example, you might put the egg on the toast and decide to have the tomatoes on the side. You might put the tomato on the toast and leave the egg to the side, or you might layer them all together. If you want to add more to this meal, try adding avocado to the toast, or herbs, spinach, or arugula to the eggs.

Lunch

Up next in your meal plan is lunch.

First, we are going to make a simple warm Salad. For this, you can steam kale, spinach, arugula, or another choice of leafy greens. Next, you are going to add tomatoes. For the dressing, you can leave it as is or choose to add a vinaigrette and olive oil mix.

Now, for protein, we are going to dive into fish. For this, you can get some anchovies and cook them in olive oil and lemon juice. The mixture can be added onto some whole wheat toast, or the toast can be kept to the side. You shouldn't add butter to your toast, but you might be able to find an olive oil spread, or you can just make extra vinaigrette dressing and dip it in there.

For some options for this meal, you can choose not to steam the greens if that doesn't appeal to you. And, if you don't like anchovies, then that's okay! Just chose another fish!

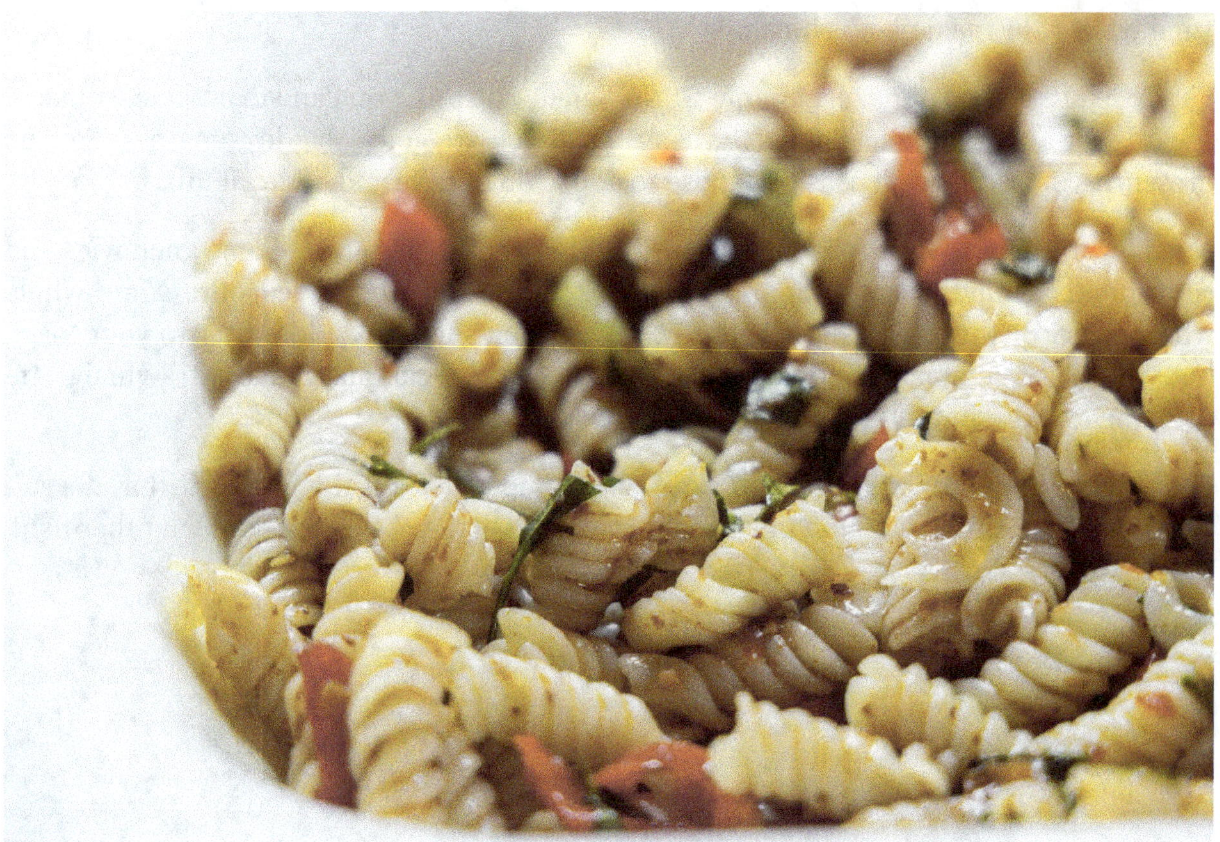

Finally, let's talk about dinner!

For this meal, you will need half a cup of whole grain pasta (any kind of noodle will do), tomato sauce (your own or store-bought), olive oil, and assorted vegetables. If you like it, you can also grab a tablespoon of parmesan cheese.

First, make pasta as you normally would! Combine the noodles and sauce together and top it with cheese. Then, do what you wish with the vegetables! You can steam them, grill them, stir fry them, or just eat them raw!

Here you have choices on what type of noodles you have, and while tomato sauce is recommended, you can get any kind you like. If you want to spice it up, add some herbs!

Day 2

Breakfast

For this one, get a slice of whole wheat toast, then some cheese (preferably a soft one such as goat's cheese, ricotta, brie, cottage cheese, or mozzarella), and either some figs or some berries of your choice.

This is something that you can layer, or you can choose to eat each separately.

Lunch

For this lunch, get a bag of mixed legume beans (or cans, I won't judge), and mix them together! Once you have completed this step add some spices and herbs. You can add garlic, basil, oregano, paprika, or whatever your heart desires.

Next, get some arugula, spinach, or kale together! Add some tomatoes, cucumbers, feta cheese, and an olive oil dressing to it!

Feel free with these meals to bring in anything you like and take out anything you don't!

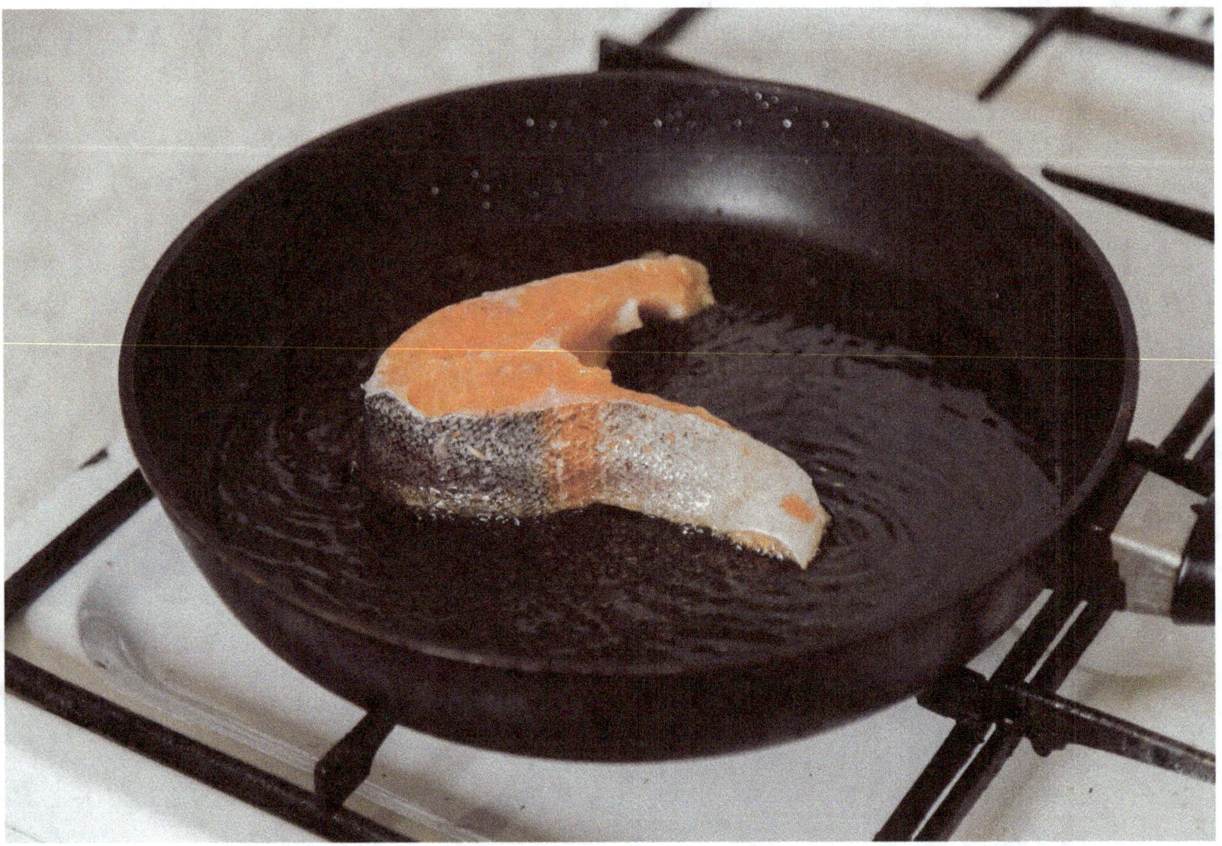

I absolutely love how hearty this meal is, while still being perfectly Mediterranean.

First, get a serving of the fish of your choice (I usually prefer salmon). Cook this by either baking, grilling, or frying, and take this time to add the herbs and spices of your choice!

Next, choose some potatoes. You can either do one big one or a few smaller ones. glaze them in olive oil and either bake them or set them on the grill.

Day 3

Breakfast

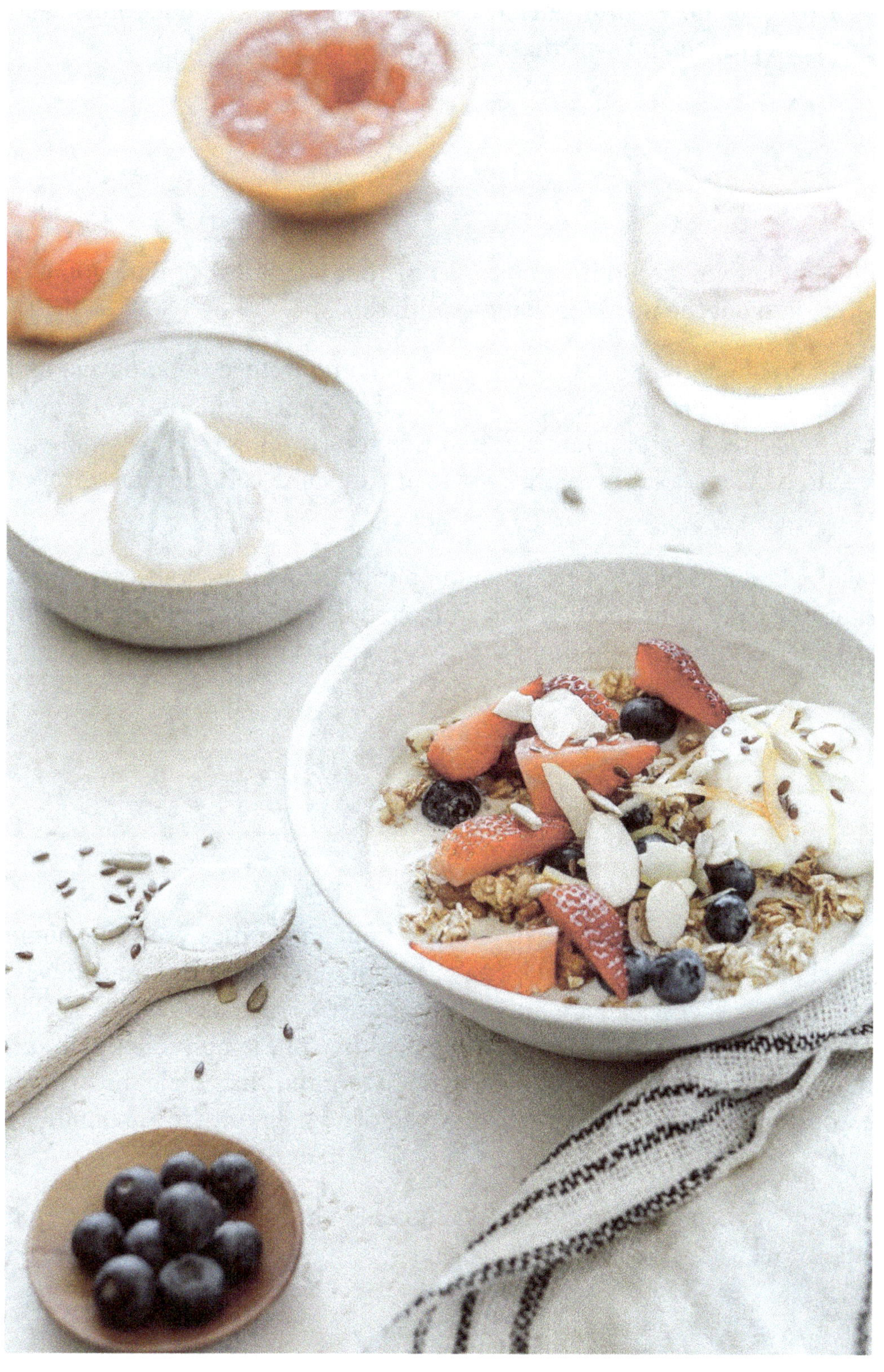

For this one, we are going to have some yogurt! Get some greek yogurt (preferably low-fat or nonfat yogurt) and the fruit of your choice. Personally, I like to add berries to my yogurt. Finally, you can add some nutty granola to your yogurt as well. If you aren't sure if your granola is a part of the Mediterranean diet, try adding some oats, nuts, and honey! This will add both crunch and sweetness to your breakfast!

Lunch

This lunch is really simple to make, so if you have a day that you know you are going to be busy, feel free to switch out the meal for that day with this one.

First, you're going to create a greek salad. Get some romaine lettuce, feta, olives, and tomatoes, along with a vinaigrette dressing. Mix it all together and put it in your container for lunch. Feel free to add a few herbs to this too! If it's a busy day and you know you are going to be using a lot of energy, you can add some cod, chicken, or even tofu to this!

Along with the salad, get some pita bread and some hummus! This will also put some energy and some protein into your food! If you want to spice this up, try an olive-oil-based hummus or some red or orange hummus.

Dinner

For this dinner, we are going to make a salad–with a little extra kick!

First, for the salad, get some kale, spinach, arugula, and romaine lettuce. Next, get some vegetables of your choice. I like to add red onion, cucumbers, tomatoes, and olives. Finally, get some shredded cheese. Personally, I will add feta crumbles or mozzarella. For the dressing, mix together some plain greek yogurt, olive oil, lemon juice, salt and pepper, garlic, and a couple of herbs of your choice. Keep in mind that while this will up your dairy intake, you can use a dressing like this instead of a vinaigrette if you don't like that type of dressing.

Finally, for protein, find some packaged smoked salmon at your local store and put that on top of the salad! Enjoy!

Day 4

Breakfast

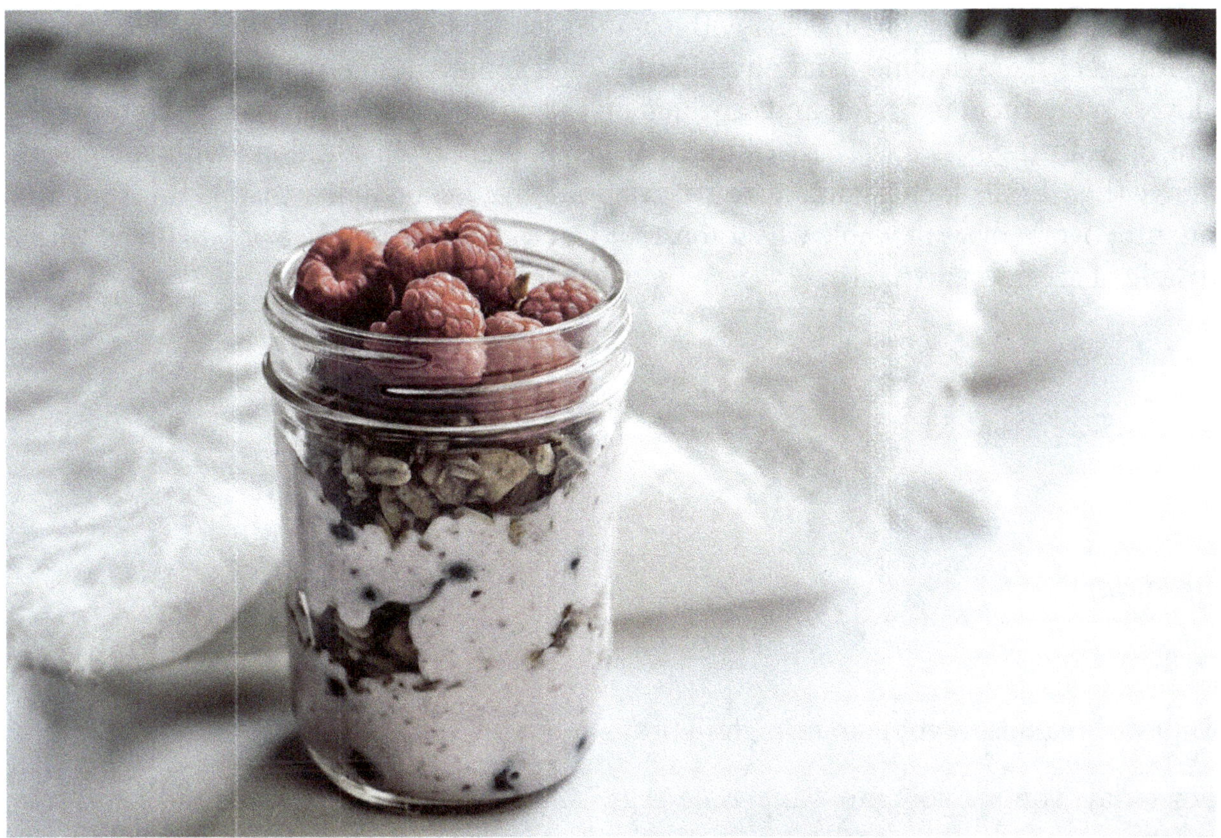

If you aren't a morning person, then this is one you will really like! We're going to make overnight oats! Find a jar or container, add half a cup of oats and half a cup of low fat milk and let that sit overnight. Next, we're going to add fruit. You can add this the night before, have it chopped up to add in the morning, or you can just make it when you wake up. I try to add at least two fruits. I will add either strawberries and bananas, black and blueberries, or both red and green apples with cinnamon. If you want to sweeten this, you can add stevia, agave syrup, or honey!

Lunch

For this lunch, you're going to need brown rice, sun-dried tomatoes, red onion, some green peas, a few herbs, black and red kidney beans, and some sliced avocado. Cook the brown rice and add your vegetables in! If you want to add a little more flavor to it, feel free to add some soy sauce. For a dose of healthy fat, add the sliced avocado to the top!

Dinner

For this meal, we're going to start with some artichoke hearts. Take two small artichoke hearts, coat them in lemon and olive oil, then add some salt and pepper and a few garlic cloves. Wrap them in tin foil and set them on the grill until they have a soft texture (you can unwrap them to check. Next, in a pan, cook some spinach along with some leafy herbs (like basil, for example). You can add some lemon juice to this and put this mixture over a piece of whole wheat toast, or you can add it to a slice of pita bread with a drizzle of greek yogurt sauce.

Day 5

Breakfast

Today's breakfast is going to be high in protein, but lower in calories!

For today, you are going to want some eggs, some sliced peppers, some salsa and sour cream, a whole wheat tortilla, and some herbs of your choice! You can also add some feta to this if you wish!

First, slice your bell peppers and cook them in a pan until they are softer in texture. Next, scramble the eggs. Once these are both cooked, add the eggs and peppers to your tortilla and top it with sour cream, salsa, and feta! To spice this up, you can add some herbs like rosemary or basil, and you can add some sliced avocado.

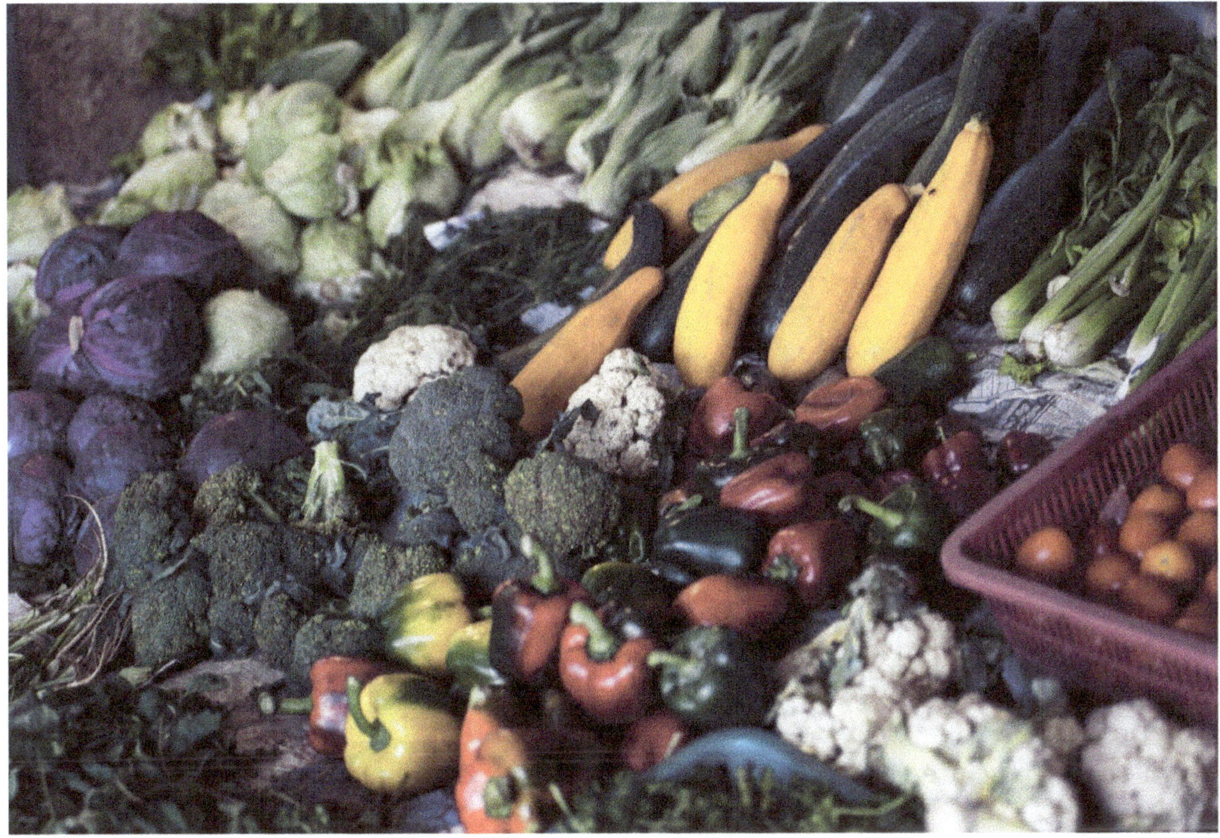

For lunch today, we are going to start with a medley of vegetables! Add in some tomatoes, cucumbers, peppers, red onion, spinach, carrots, lettuce, and whatever else you wish. Also, we are adding leafy greens, this isn't a traditional salad. Chop the leaves up finely and add them in the same proportion as all of the other vegetables.

Once you have your mix made, set it aside and take out a chicken breast. You can season this with salt and pepper, garlic, oregano, thyme, and lemon juice. Cook in a pan with olive oil, and once it's done, chop it up and add it to your food! Once you finish this step, you can either add olive oil vinaigrette to it or add a greek-yogurt-based dressing!

Dinner

For dinner, let's start with a serving of fish! For this, feel free to choose cod, halibut, tuna, salmon, or whatever else you might fancy. Spice this up with salt, pepper, garlic, lemon juice, and olive oil. Then, wrap it in tin foil and you can either set it on the grill or in the oven. The next thing you're going to want is some brown rice. Cook a small portion and then add it to a bowl. Next, add some spinach and arugula to a bowl along with some tomatoes. Drizzle it and the rice in olive oil and vinaigrette dressing. Once your fish is done, add it to the top! This bowl should be delicious and filling!

Day 6

Breakfast

Now we are going to do another greek yogurt option, this time with a more tropical twist. Personally, I find that plain greek yogurt is best for this one as it is best to help you taste all of the flavors we are going to add. For adding fruit to this yogurt, we are going to add some things that might not be in every person's fruit drawer. Think of adding some mango or kiwi, or pineapple to your bowl! Once you've chosen your fruit, add some nuts, oats, or a granola mix. Finally, add some honey to it to make it sweet!

This breakfast will have protein and essential nutrients. It's easy, and if you want to cut down on morning prep time, you can cut up your fruit the night before!

Lunch

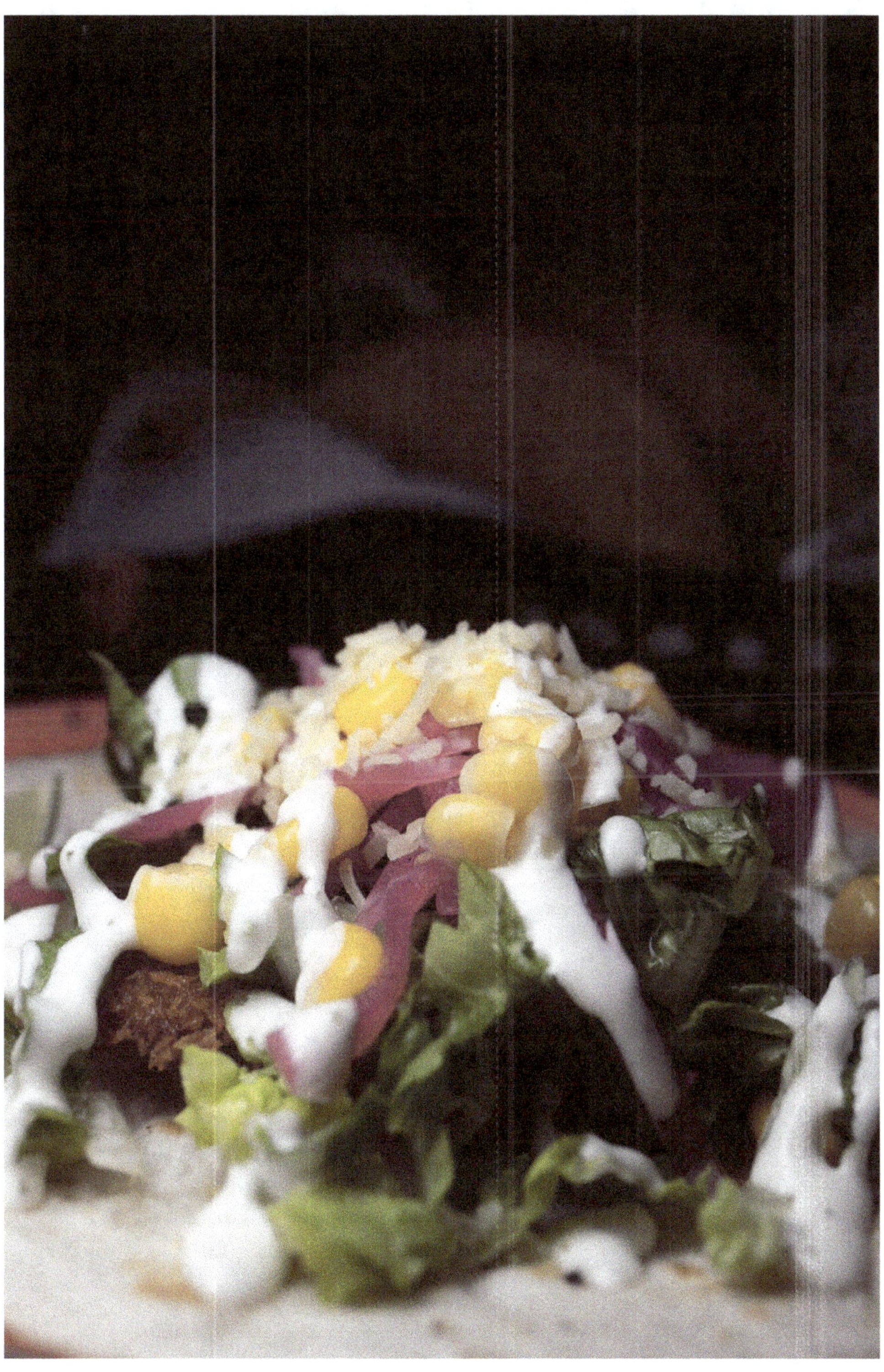

Wraps are always a win for lunch! So,let's make one!

For this wrap, get some white fish (cod or halibut), lettuce, tomatoes, onions, and peppers! The fish can be made the night before if you would like! Simply use some salt, pepper, garlic, lemon juice, and herbs to spice this up! If you want to try a different spice mix, feel free to!

Next, you can choose what you would like for your sauce! I love using a greek yogurt sauce for this recipe, but you can also use sour cream and salsa for a different–but amazing flavor!

Dinner

We're making another bowl! For this one, you can either start with brown rice or some romaine lettuce.

Now for the topping, let's get a collection of vegetables. Get some tomatoes, mushrooms, potatoes, zucchini, squash, peppers, onions, carrots, and other vegetables you want to add! Coat all of this in some salt, pepper, and olive oil. Then, put it in a baking dish and set it in your oven. Once this finishes cooking, add it over top of your base, and you are finished!

Day 7

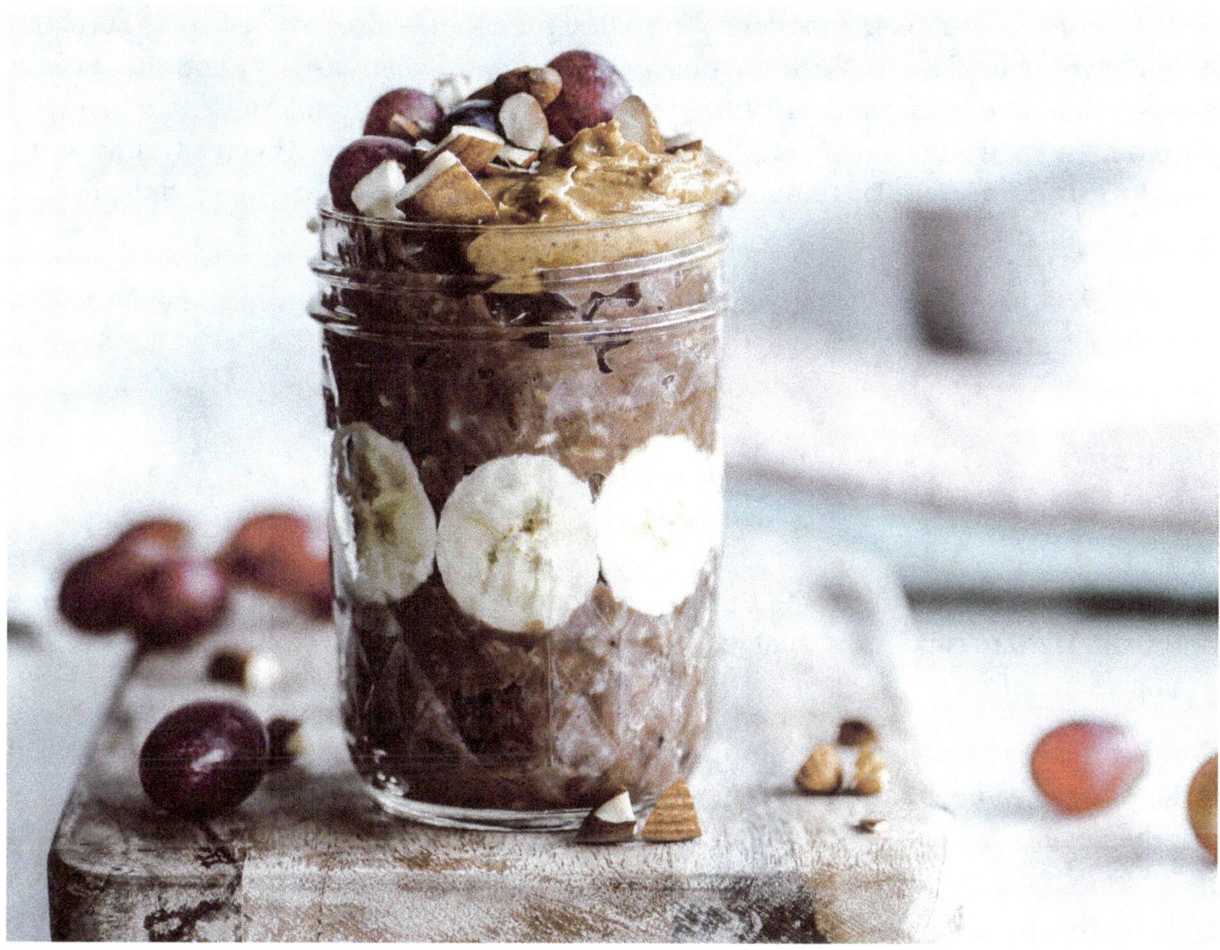

You have made it to the end of the week my friend! And it is time for a reward! Remember, The Mediterranean doesn't eliminate sweets, or really any food group! It just limits the ideal quantity.

For this last meal, we are going to start with a base of oats! If you can do these warm, it works better with this recipe, but it can still be done with overnight oats if needed! For warm oats, you can do a single serving in the microwave at a one-to-one ratio (one cup of water for every cut of oats).

Once you have your oats, add some cocoa powder, a banana, and some dark chocolate chips. Together, this combination can provide you with energy and satisfy a sweet tooth!

Lunch

For this lunch, we are going to make some zucchini noodles. To start, get some zucchini. If you have a spiralizer, you can then make them into noodles easily! If not, that's okay! just take a potato peeler and use it to create slices of zucchini. Cook these in a pan with olive oil, and you will have a nice al dente texture. Once you have this ready, add some tomato sauce, mozzarella, tomatoes, peppers, onions, and either some white fish or some shrimp or clam.

All of these ingredients together will give you delicious pasta whilst being full of vegetables and protein.

Dinner

For our final meal, we are going to make a Mediterranean-style pizza. First, find some flatbread. If there isn't any available, then try some pita bread! It's often the perfect size for a personal pizza.

For this recipe, you can make your own sauce using tomatoes and herbs (which is typical in Mediterranean regions). To do this, boil your tomatoes so that you can take the skins off, then combine them with some olive oil, minced onions, and your choices of herbs. If it's chunky, that's perfectly fine! Alternatively, you can also use the leftover sauce from your lunch!

Once you have your sauce, spread it over the flatbread and add some spinach, basil, mozzarella, tomatoes, red onion, and any other vegetables you want to add! While many American pizzas do come covered in cheese, here you will actually be leaving some sauce exposed. Add the vegetables first, then take a brick of mozzarella and cut it into slices. Place the slices on your pizza, and then let it bake! Once it's done, you can add some arugula to the top!

All of these meals don't have to be eaten in this exact order. They can be mixed, matched, and substituted as needed! This can give you some ideas for future recipes and help you to see what you might do for your meals in the future! Maybe you'll find some favorite recipes here!

Chapter 4: Potential Benefits of the Mediterranean Diet

Traditionally, when a new diet joins the mainstream diet culture world, it's been created by someone, or a group of people, who have spent a bit of time learning about nutrition, and a lot of time online marketing or influencing others. The creator of many of the diets we see may have a degree in nutritional science or a related field, or they might be a doctor, though not necessarily in a nutrition-based field. A lot of these diets focus on a tiny part of the human body and ignore the negative side effects that they can bring to the rest. Now, why is it important to make this distinction?

Simply put, this is who you tell that even if you've tried other diets and had them negatively affect your health, you should still absolutely try the Mediterranean diet.

As we mentioned in a previous chapter, the Mediterranean diet is a cultural eating pattern. It's one that people took interest in when we realized that while most of the developed world seemed to be suffering from heart issues and other diseases, this area wasn't.

This diet was found by chance, not created by someone who saw a marketing opportunity. It has decades of research behind it, meaning that we can rely on the information I'm going to share with you below. And, my favorite part about this is that it's already followed around the world by people who share what it's like, so if you are curious, there is a community out there that has been there for all of those decades (and even centuries). Now, when we take a look at people who follow this diet and compare them to people who follow an average diet, what do we see?

The Health of Your Heart Improves

Your heart is one of the most important organs in your body. With that in mind, let me give you some statistics that the Center for Disease Control (CDC) in America has given us.

Heart disease is an unbiased killer. Whether you are a man, woman, caucasian, African American, Latinx, or a part of another group, it doesn't matter. It's the number one killer of all adults. Every 34 seconds, heart disease takes a life. In 2020, that cost us

697,000 lives. This has been linked to our diet time and time again. It's not uncommon for someone not to eat any fruits or vegetables in a day. Red meat is the cornerstone of so many meals in the average American diet, and it's a regular part of the menu in many other countries as well. We all also eat things with extremely high-fat content.

Furthermore, many people work extremely busy schedules. Because of this, they tend to rely more on fast food products to keep them going rather than on making food. So many things are added to fast food to boost the taste, and these things can throw off your hormones, gut health, and heart health so fast. In addition to that, because they are loaded with these things, they contain way more calories than they should, and as a result, they add a ton of weight to your body! Notably, this is more of a problem in America because there aren't many restrictions on what can be added to food. You should check your country's guidelines to see what they say.

The beautiful thing about the Mediterranean diet is that it developed outside of all of these practices. Their natural environment allowed the people of this region to avoid so many of these issues.

Your heart has to pump through all of the food you put into your body. It plays a role in processing what you eat and turning it into things that your body can use. The Mediterranean diet will aid it in this effort rather than filling it with chemicals and hormones that will further hurt you.

Your Cardiovascular System

Your cardiovascular system includes your entire circulatory system for your blood, and that means your heart too!

The typical diet hurts the heart by increasing blood pressure and cholesterol. Cholesterol is essentially tiny fat deposits that are circulating through your blood. You are supposed to have at least some cholesterol, as the fat helps to protect your cells. However, if you have too much, and run out of cells for the fat to protect, then you have free fat essentially floating around in your blood. Again, a small amount is okay.

If you have a large amount of this fat in your body, then it can group together and get stuck along a wall in your circulatory system. If a tiny bit gets stuck, it starts to act like a magnet. It brings more fat. Eventually, these fat deposits can start to restrict the blood flow going by. If they get big enough, they can block this area completely. Now, if this happens near your arms or legs, you will be in pain, and if it's not treated, you could lose the limb. If it happens near any major organs or inhibits blood flow to an organ, it will hurt the function of that organ and cause it to stop working. The organ could fail if this is left untreated.

On this list of organs is the heart. If the heart can pump blood, it will stop beating and cause a heart attack.

As scary as that sounds, your brain is also an organ that could be affected by this. If a blockage like this happens within your brain, the part of the brain that is dealing with the block will shut down. Eventually, this will result in a stroke.

The Mediterranean diet can help. First of all, the recommended eating pattern keeps your cholesterol levels low, so you don't have to worry about most of these issues in the first place. Second of all, if there is nothing being added to those buildups of cholesterol, they will eventually break apart, be processed by the body, and fade from existence, leaving your blood circulatory system clean!

Diabetes and Related Disease

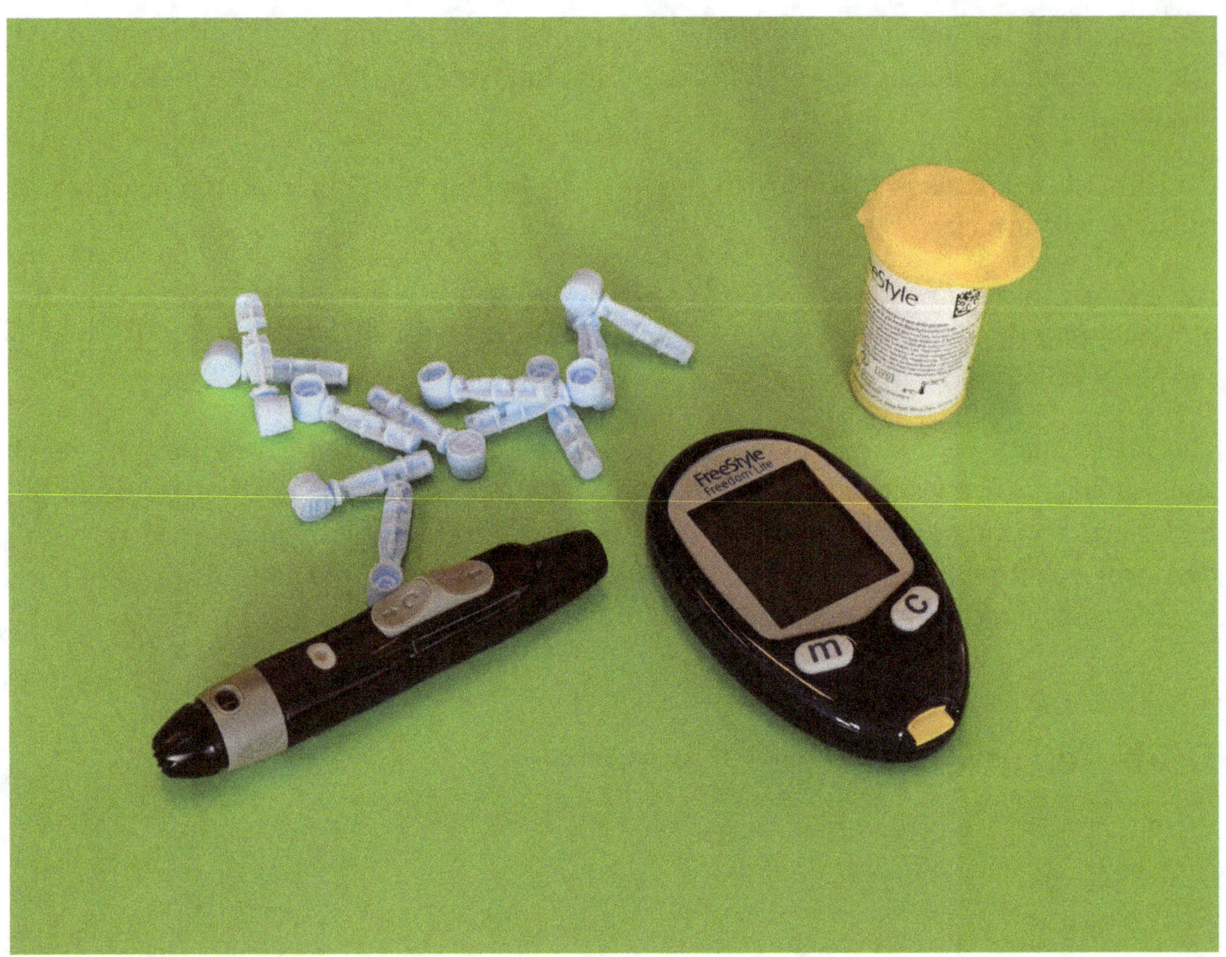

All of the issues with food that we talked about in the previous section come with another issue. In the diet, there are a lot of things that will raise a person's blood sugar levels. If insulin production runs into any issues, it will result in diabetes. Diabetes has been further linked to Alzheimer's many times.

The Mediterranean diet can help with this. It's often recommended as a diet for those with diabetes because it can help keep blood sugar levels down. Fruits and vegetables add a ton of necessary vitamins and minerals to the diet without raising your blood sugar. The foods that you eat won't be high in calories for the most part, and the fat content isn't too high, except for things like olive oil which won't harm your blood sugar levels. Stable blood sugar levels, even when you already have diabetes, can lead to the prevention of Alzheimers.

Protects Brain Function

There are a couple of ways this happens. First of all, our brains do require fuel from our bodies, and they can only take the fuel we give them. As such, when that fuel is loaded with fat, sugar, chemicals, hormones, and preservatives, it all goes to the brain and gets stuck there. It hurts our ability to do our daily tasks. Now, once we start with something like the Mediterranean diet, our body has a chance to circle all of these toxins out of our body!

Second, the food will promote your brain's function. Not only are we flushing your brain off the toxic chemicals, but we are replacing those with vital nutrients that will help your brain work better in the long run! This will help improve your thinking and focus, and it can help you think smarter in the long run!

Helps With Sleep

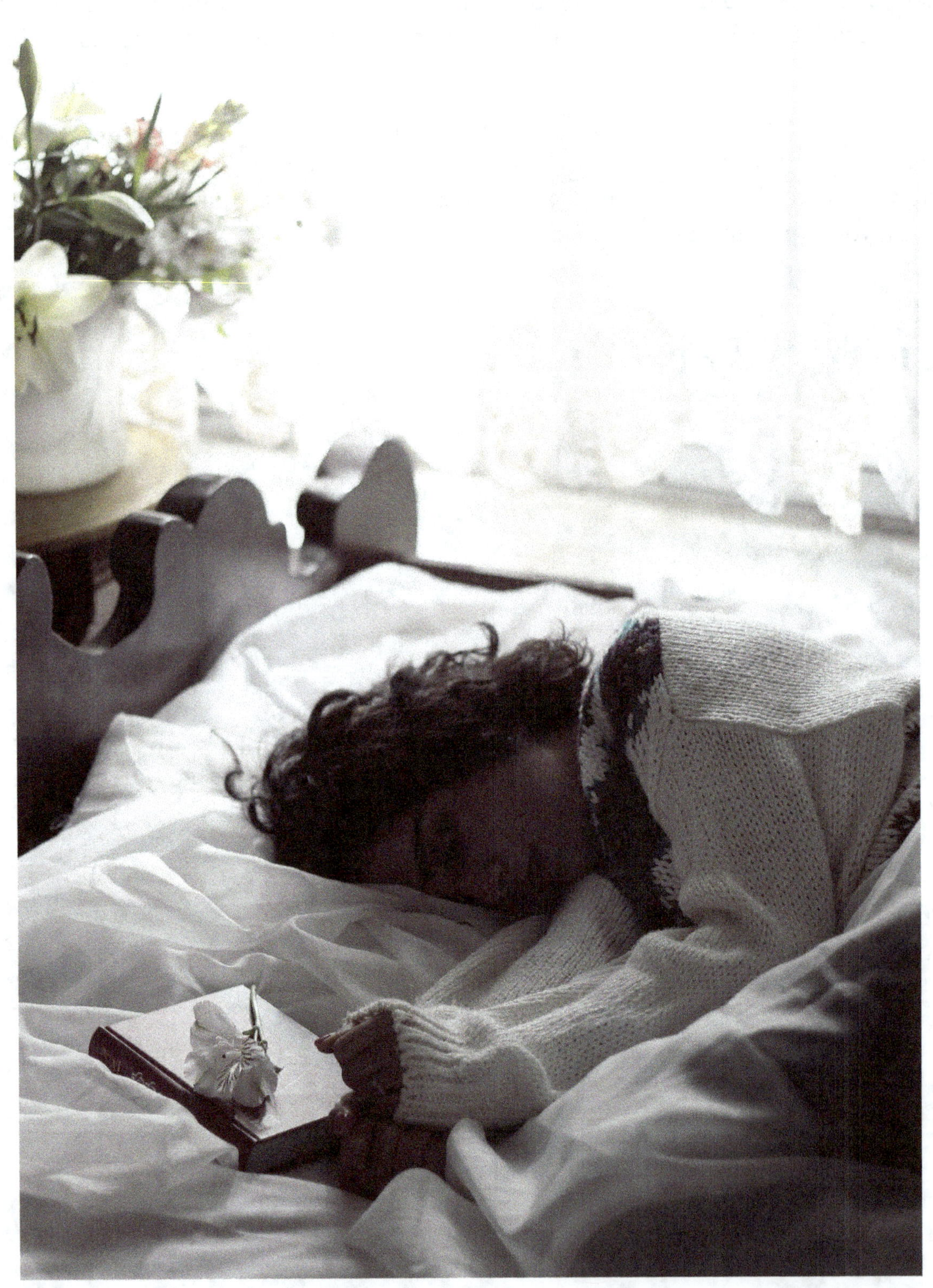

The sugar that we take in, as well as all of the hormones and harmful objects from our food, come together to wreak havoc on our sleep cycle. Not only do those toxic hormones and chemicals wreak havoc on the brain's ability to think and function, but it also messes with the circadian rhythm, which controls how sleepy we are. Typically, it can cause our body to throw off the wrong signal at the wrong time. The Mediterranean diet helps to re-balance and fix those signals so that you will end up sleeping better!

Improvements to Your Mood

As you might imagine, hormones that are strong enough to impact your sleep cycle can absolutely have an impact on your mood too! Once the work is done by the Mediterranean diet to re-balance your body, you should see things like your personal happiness, your feelings of contentment, and your ability to endure difficult situations all increase while more negative emotions will decrease.

Weight Loss

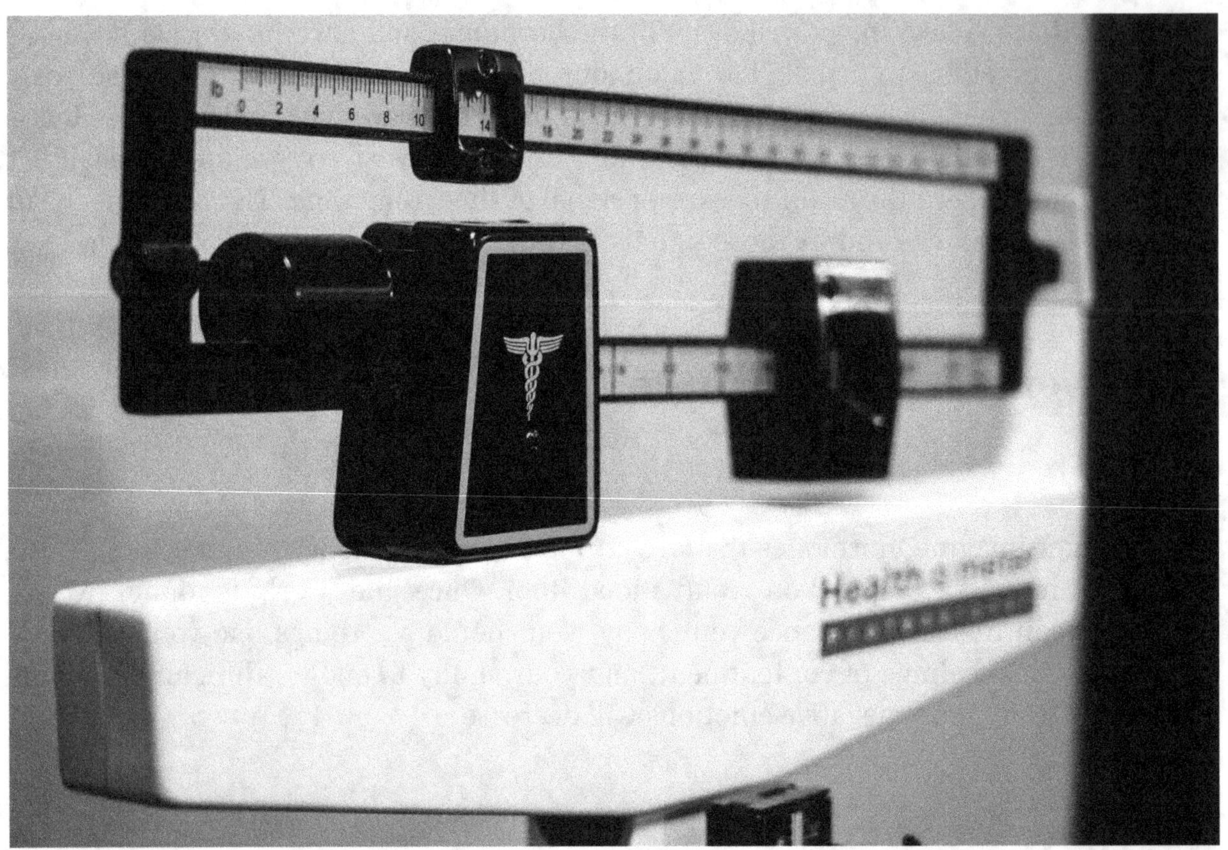

Let's be honest, this is why a lot of us generally intend to start a new diet. We want to lose weight. Now, I've included this benefit last to show you all of the amazing things that the Mediterranean diet can do for you that don't just include weight loss. That being said, I know that it might be one of the major reasons you have picked up this book. So, let's dive into this. Yes, the Mediterranean diet can help with weight loss, but it might not be a quick process. The weight you lose will naturally come from a healthy diet rather than another method. To show you what I mean, let's take a look at some popular diets to see how they help with weight loss and how they affect you.

Chapter 5: Diets That Will Help You Lose Weight

If there is one thing I want you to be able to do by the time you read this book, it's to make an informed decision. You cannot easily do so without having all of the knowledge. So, I will now present you with the facts on some other diets that also help you lose weight.

Atkins Diet

The Atkins diet relies on very little carbs (under 20 grams a day) and much more protein to help you lose weight. Studies show that it works, and it works quickly. With the Atkins diet, many people approach their goal weight quickly, with some losing five pounds in their first week alone. This, when compared to other diets, is phenomenal. Additionally, it can lower blood sugar and pressure levels. With this diet, you add more carbs back into your diet as you get closer to your ideal weight.

Now, the Atkins diet relies heavily on meat, which can be full of fat. This can increase your cholesterol and lead to you being more likely to develop heart disease. Because you add your barbs back in, you're likely to level off your weight loss eventually, and once you start eating normally again, you'll regain your weight, and potentially gain even more than you had when you started.

HCG

The HCG diet can make you lose weight even faster than Atkins. You might lose up to two pounds a day. Now, how is this done?

First, you start by taking HCG supplements. These are hormones that are secreted during pregnancy. They fool your body into thinking you are pregnant, causing shifts in your calorie use as your body prepares for a baby. During this time, you eat a 500-calorie diet, which your body will utilize only for its essential functions. It will burn fat for everyone, causing you to lose weight. Doctors caution against this diet. There are no documented benefits, but if you have chronic health conditions or have ever struggled with an eating disorder in your past, it's extremely dangerous for you to try this diet.

Extreme Low-Fat Diet

Now, in theory, this diet sounds amazing. Even the Mediterranean diet recommends low-fat products.

Now, our diet commonly consists of about 30% of our calories coming from fat (Bjarnadottir, 2019). Now, to achieve this, the diet cuts out nearly all animal-based products including meat, eggs, and dairy. As such, protein ends up only making up about ten to twenty percent of your diet. The rest is carb based.

For those who have fast morbid obesity, this diet can bring about a rapid change and it can cause nearly 150 pounds of weight loss on average. This diet has amazing benefits for those with heart disease, type 2 diabetes, and multiple sclerosis.

Now, fat is important to our body. If you remember, in a previous section we talked about the importance of having some cholesterol to protect cells within the body. A diet this low in fat makes that very hard to maintain. Furthermore, it's very easy to develop a very unhealthy diet with this plan. Your body craves things that aren't good for it, and as a result, it causes you to eat foods that are in the diet but not good for you.

Vegan Diets

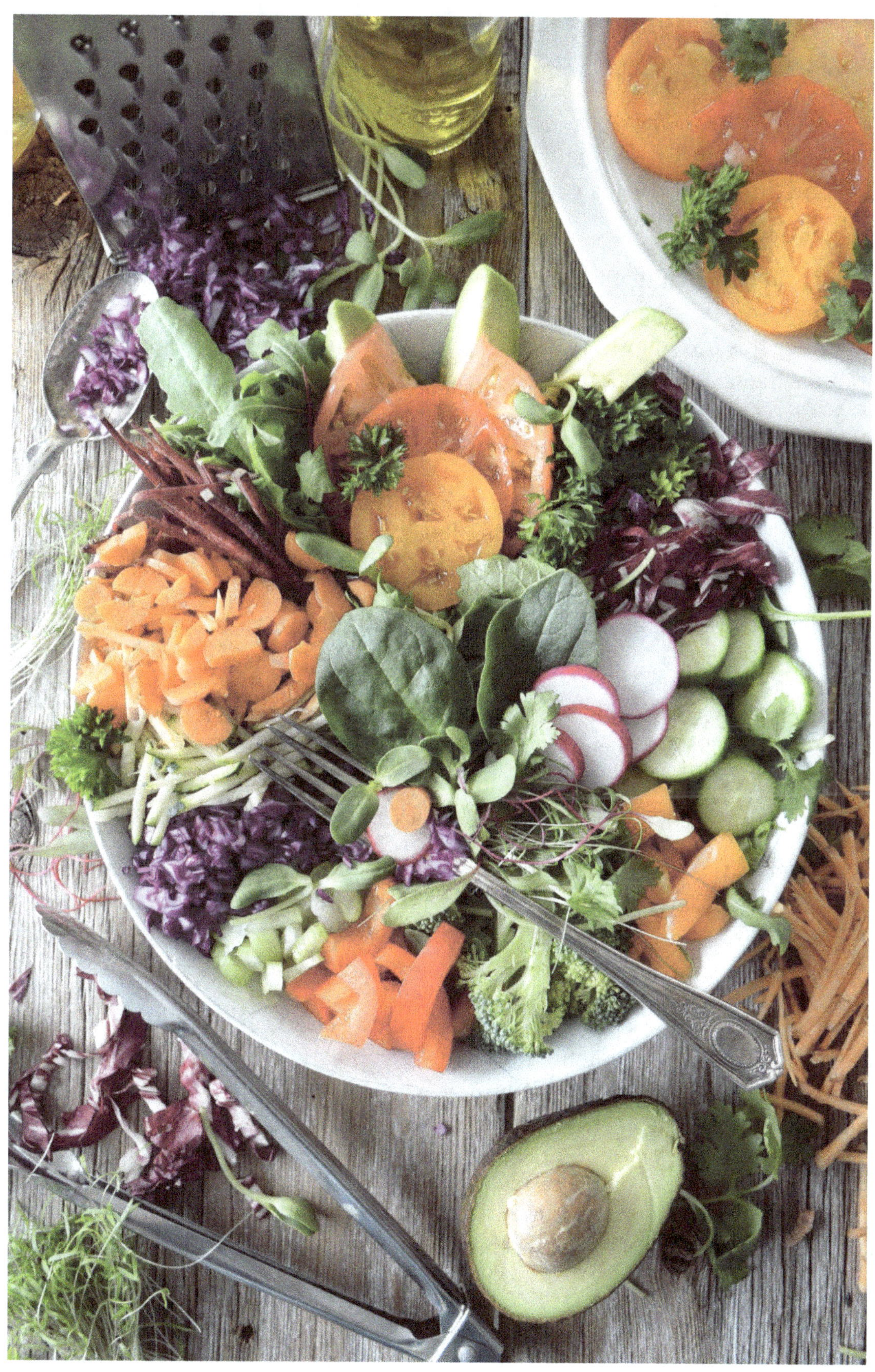

These are getting more and more popular as time goes on. Vegan diets exclude anything made from an animal. To get protein, they tend to rely on things like beans, and soy-based products.

Vegan diets can help with weight loss, although they aren't as helpful as some other methods. Additionally, it helps with heart disease and diabetes management, and it can help with brain power.

That being said, a vegan diet can be expensive. Because you aren't eating any meat, you aren't getting some of the vitamins that you need that are essential to your health. In order to make this up, you will need to buy either vitamin-enriched foods or a long list of the vitamins themselves, both of which are costly.

Paleo

Paleo's origins trace themselves back to the paleolithic era and rely on a similar eating pattern.

In previous chapters, we've mentioned that there are a lot of difficulties associated with the processing of foods, including added chemicals and toxins that harm us. The Mediterranean region gets out of this because their food sources are so well used that they don't have nearly as much processing to do.

The paleo diet uses another method. It brings us back to the time before processed food was really a thing. You rely on foods that don't need any processing in order to be made. This means all fruit, vegetables, and non-processed meat is available to you, but most carbs and all processed items are not. This does include dairy products as well.

Paleo is promoted as a clean way of eating, and it seems to be. It can help sharpen mental focus, and provide benefits for heart diseases and type two diabetes. That being said, carbs are an important part of our diet. You may feel lethargic on this diet and you may face issues with low blood sugar because of this. Grains also contain some vitamins and minerals that we need so we now have to find an alternate way to get those.

Lastly, because this is a severe elimination diet, you run the risk of developing allergies to the foods you aren't eating and becoming ill when you do try to consume processed foods.

Keto

Keto is a cross between paleo and Atkins. It also focuses on non-processed clean eating, with a limit of 25 grams of carbs per day. As you might imagine, keto comes with a lot of similar benefits, such as lower blood pressure and blood sugar, and a level of mental clarity that comes from the lack of processed foods.

Keto is high fat and as such it raises your cholesterol, risk of heart disease, and chances of developing allergies later in life. The high-fat content can hurt your liver and kidneys, and if you face issues with hypoglycemia it can make it worse. It has also been reported that keto can cause hypoglycemia.

Intermittent Fasting

Intermittent fasting doesn't limit what you can eat. It limits when you can eat it. For this diet, there is a period when you eat and a period when you don't. Now, this can help you lose weight and it can help with sleep, blood pressure, and heart issues. It can both help and hurt diabetes sufferers, and someone with diabetes may need to be willing to break their fast if they have low blood sugar.

Now, this diet can cause hypoglycemia to develop. Its strict calorie counting can also lead to the development of an eating disorder.

If a person already has these issues, they should not partake in this diet.

Raw Food Diet

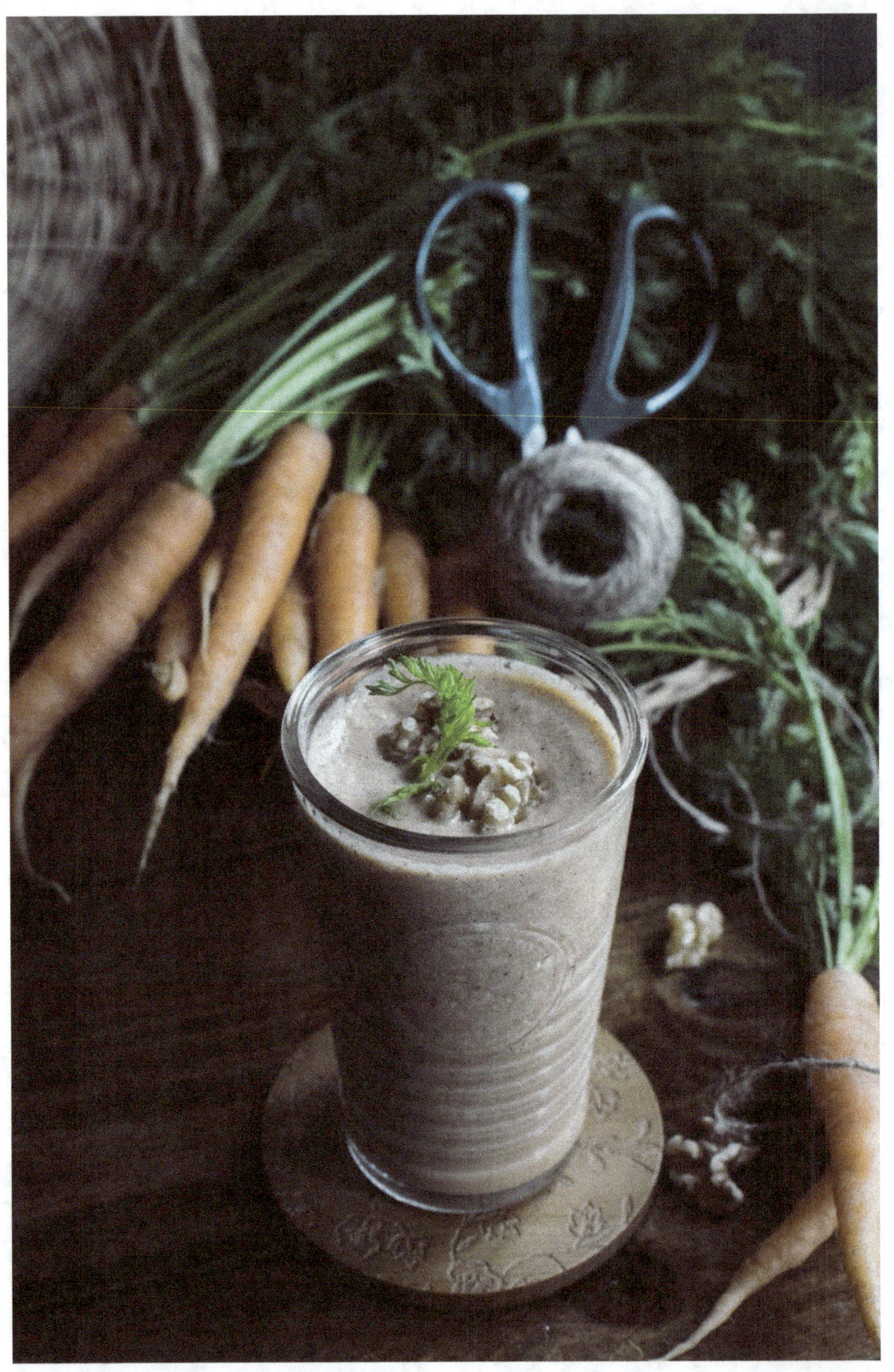

This diet is a bit different. As you might tell by the title, there is very little cooking involved. You are eating raw fruits and vegetables, nuts and seeds, sushi, and some raw eggs. Some grains are a part of this diet too. This diet is native to India and has shown to help with weight loss as it very much limits what you can consume. Other than weight loss, not many benefits have been recorded, but there are risks to this diet for anyone with a health condition, as well as children and the elderly.

If any of these diets caught your attention, feel free to follow up on more information for them. You don't necessarily have to follow them in full either, as you might be able to incorporate some elements of the diet that you like into the Mediterranean diet. For example, I like to take the paleo element of having as little processed food as possible and making it a part of my dietary structure. You can also add practices like intermittent fasting to the diet.

Chapter 6: Mediterranean Weight Loss Journey

One of the things that drew researchers to the Mediterranean region is the fact that many of the people there aren't suffering from weight issues. In many developed countries, at least one third of the population is obese, and as many as two third of the population is overweight. These numbers are harrowing, but when we look over to the Mediterranean region, they don't seem to exist. What we are going to do next is going to help put their "why" into perspective.

Weight Maintenance With The Mediterranean Diet

Now, this region of the world is full of generally healthy people at a generally healthy weight. Those who move to the region seem to adapt to this lifestyle, and those who try this lifestyle outside of the region seem to be able to experience the benefits too, and this includes weight loss. Now, how does this happen?

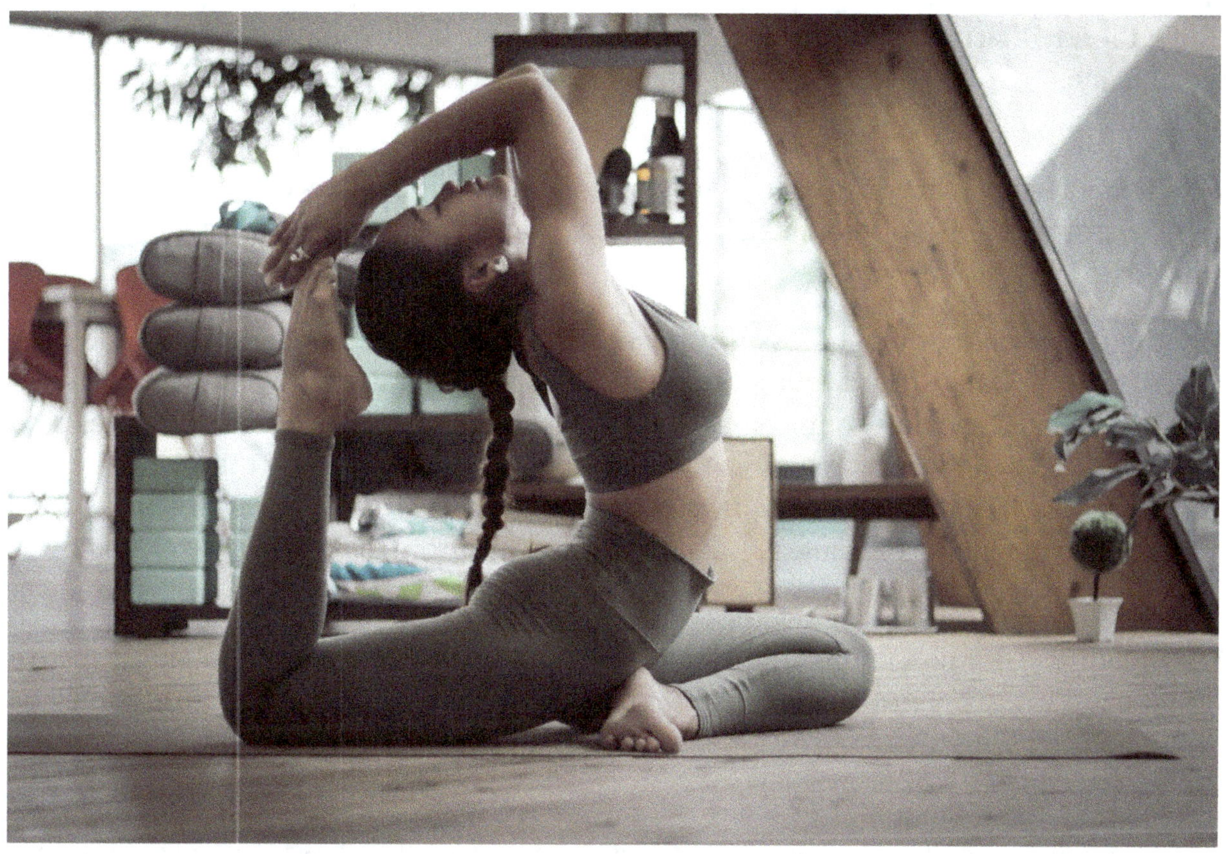

Here is what is believed to be one key component of this lifestyle's success. They live a balanced life. Many cultures favor hard work, which does accomplish a lot of things. However, a lot of science is coming and saying that working constantly isn't good for a person. A person does need to work, but they also need to be able to have time to exercise, time to see their family, time to themselves, and so on.

Stress seems to have an effect on weight gain, and not being able to have this balance does create stress.

You should absolutely fight to have this balance in your life wherever it is possible. It will go a long way in keeping you sane, and mentally able to lose weight!

The Ingredients for Weight Loss

There are a few things that go into the weight loss paradigm.

Now, one is dietary habits. These do matter quite a bit in the grand scheme of losing weight. You have to be eating the right foods. You have to be doing some calorie tracking.

Now, the Mediterranean diet food pyramid outlines a healthy eating plan pretty well. The balance that this gives you will already help out when it comes to designing your diet plan in some cases.

When it comes to managing your own calories, which will have its own section, keep in mind that there are a lot of foods out there that don't have many calories, but they will fill you up all the same.

Another major part of weight loss is exercise. It's recommended to get at least one hour of exercise per day. How you chose to do that is up to you! Even if you're just walking, you are out and moving your body. You can also bike, dance, swim, do yoga, and so much more. All of these activities work to get your body moving, and they work to burn those calories. Try not to overcompensate your workouts with food or energy bars. This will lead to you not burning any fat, and it will stop you from losing weight.

Finally, there is your overall health. Weight is just one measure of health. There is also the function of our heart, lungs, and circulatory system. There is our brain, our digestive system, our other organs, and so on. If you are facing issues with your health, it may be making it very hard for you to lose weight.

You should make it a point to have regular checkups with your doctor. It's not fun to go in when you are overweight, especially since that is often all they want to talk about, but it is important. A physical can catch issues early on, and they can help you get them fixed before the impact is long-term.

Another part of health maintenance is, again, exercise. When you exercise, you aren't just working to lose weight. You are stretching your muscles, your heart rate is rising, your lungs are working, and your body is doing a lot!

That work is all going toward keeping your body in shape. Your heart, lung, and muscle function all improve with exercise, regardless of how many calories you've had that day.

Tracking Your Calories

Now, there are doctors out there who tell you to calculate every last calorie that you take in and to make sure that you don't miss anything. This way, you know exactly what's going into your body and you can make decisions based on that data. Then, there are doctors that tell you not to do that. Doing that leads to issues with food, and for sensitive groups, it can lead to an eating disorder or at least, a relapse.

Now neither is wrong. Knowing this can help you make decisions, but if you have a history of eating disorders or you know you are sensitive about food, then it might do more harm than good. I am going to present strategies for both options, and you can choose which one you think will work best.

First, if you want to count your calories, the best way to do so is to get an app on your phone. There are apps out there today that allow you to scan a barcode of a food item. They will then give you the details of the food item so you can input how many calories were in it. From there you can make decisions on what you want to eat for the rest of the day, and you have some running data to look back at when you are making decisions or meal planning later.

Now, if you don't want to go that route (or you know you can't) there is another option to still have this data, albeit a less accurate form, and not have to worry about it everyday. Start your week with a meal plan. Lay out exactly what you intend to have. Then, you can either look online to get the total amount of calories in your dish, or you can use a similar app to scan items as you purchase them in grocery stores, and you can have your numbers there. This gives you more of a weekly calorie intake rather than a daily one.

Again, between these two options, choose the one that you think will serve you and your mental health best, and that there is a better plan for you out there than using that one!

Be Accountable for What Goes Into Your Body

One thing I love about the Mediterranean diet is that all food groups are featured on it. There really isn't anything you can't have, but it does restructure the food that you can have and it makes some big changes.

As you meal plan and work on your diet, keep in mind what you are putting in there. Does your meal plan align with the recommendations for the diet? Does it not?

Perhaps there is a lot of red meat there. Perhaps there are a lot of sweets.

I'm not here to judge. We all have weeks where we slip up. It's a bad week, and we cheer ourselves up with sweets. It's been really busy and we're eating fast food. I'm no stranger to this, and I'm sure you aren't either.

The key is to not let these things ruin your diet. When you fell off your bike as a child, you probably got right back into the saddle and started pedaling again before too long. It's time to do that here too.

First, admit that it wasn't your best week in terms of sticking to your diet. You know, even if you don't admit it to yourself, that you made a few blunders. Don't let those minor mistakes become dark secrets.

Second, plan for how you will do better next week. What new plan are you going to try? Is there anything healthy that can curb your sweet tooth? Are there any meals you can have together already for those busy days? It's up to you to find out!

Consider Your Sources of Nutrients

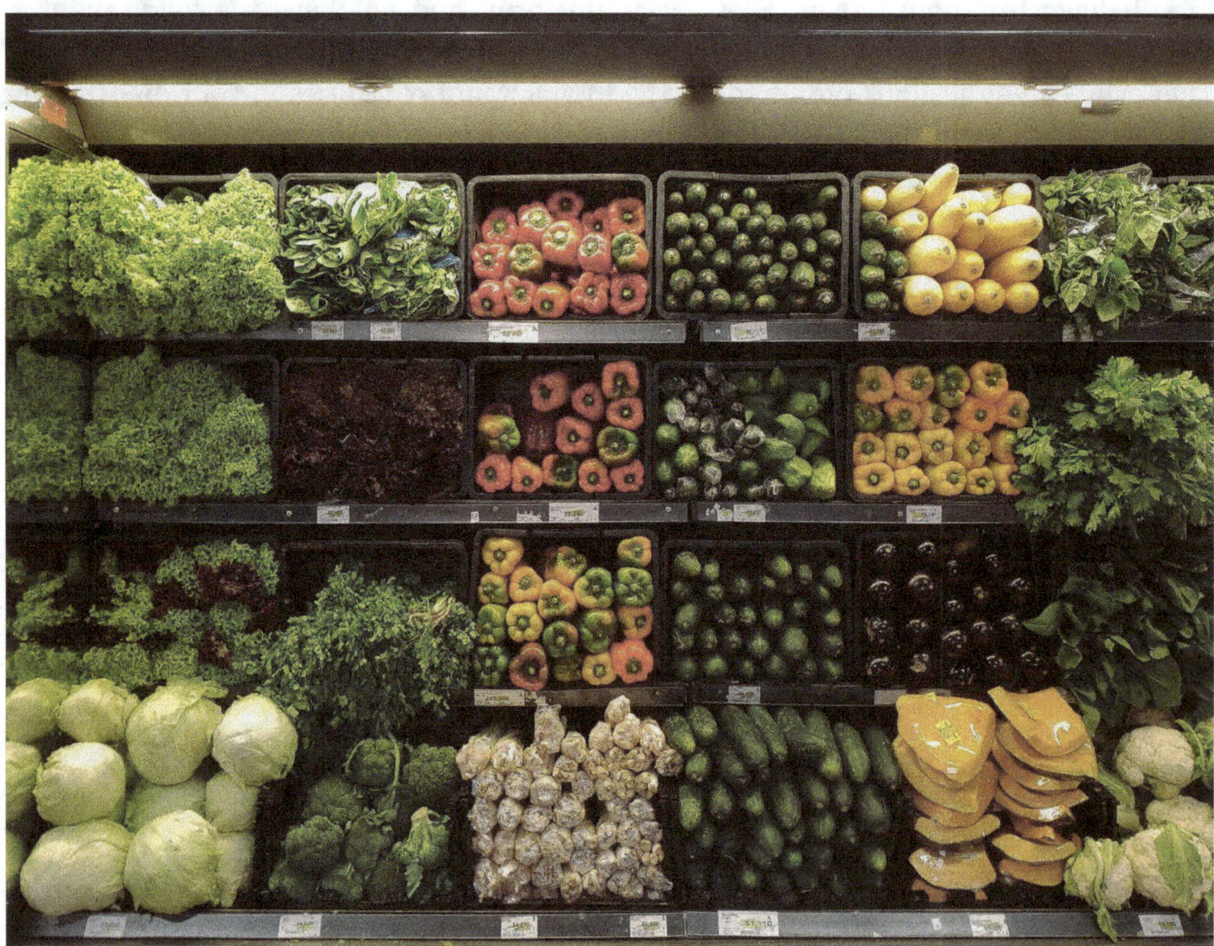

It's no secret that some foods are better for you than others. Now, let's talk about that a little more when it comes to the Mediterranean diet.

First, let's discuss protein. The Mediterranean diet relies primarily on fish and beans and a little bit of white meat in order to help you get the protein that you need. When it comes to weight loss, some options will be better for you. It's safe to say that organic is the way to go when you can, as it won't have any hormones or chemicals that are toxic to your body. You should stay away from processed meat and fish. While it might be more convenient, these are loaded up with these toxic materials, and as a result, you might find that you have more unnecessary calories in your food.

Now, for vegetables. You should take the same things into consideration. When possible, fresh vegetables are better than canned ones. If you are worried about your vegetables going bad, try freezing them. For those on a tight budget, many vegetables can be bought frozen, and they often don't have much processing done to them.

Up next is fruit. The same information in the vegetable section applies to fruit as well, but there are a few things to add. Some fruits are better than others. If you are trying to lose weight, then berries such as strawberries, blueberries, blackberries, and raspberries along with citrus fruits, are going to help you more.

Finally, let's talk about carbohydrates. First, whole grain carbs are the ones that you want.

Second, let's think of carbs in terms of weight loss. If you are aiming to lose weight, consider cutting your carb intake back to about two to three times a week, and only having them for one meal on that day. Diets that reduce your overall carb intake have been proven to help with weight loss (although, unlike the Mediterranean, they rarely offer other benefits). If we can implement that practice into the Mediterranean diet, then we can lose weight faster.

Keeping You Full

Now, one way we're going to lose weight is if we make sure that we stay full even though we have a low-calorie budget.

For this, we rely on low-calorie foods. It probably comes as no surprise that vegetables are on the list. If we are trying to get less calories into our day while still eating enough food to feel satisfied, then we should aim to eat less carbohydrates.

More protein from sources like beans and soy-based products can also help us stay full for longer periods of time.

When we talk about weight loss, I don't want you to feel like you have to do it because your doctor said it or because everyone else is telling you to lose weight. I want you to do it for yourself.

Weight loss can be a struggle for a lot of people. So, may I present to you a list of motivations that can help you remind you why it's important to lose weight rather than relying on the worlds of others for motivation?

Benefits of Weight Loss

Other than the "weight loss" part of weight loss, what's so good about it?

Lowers Blood Pressure

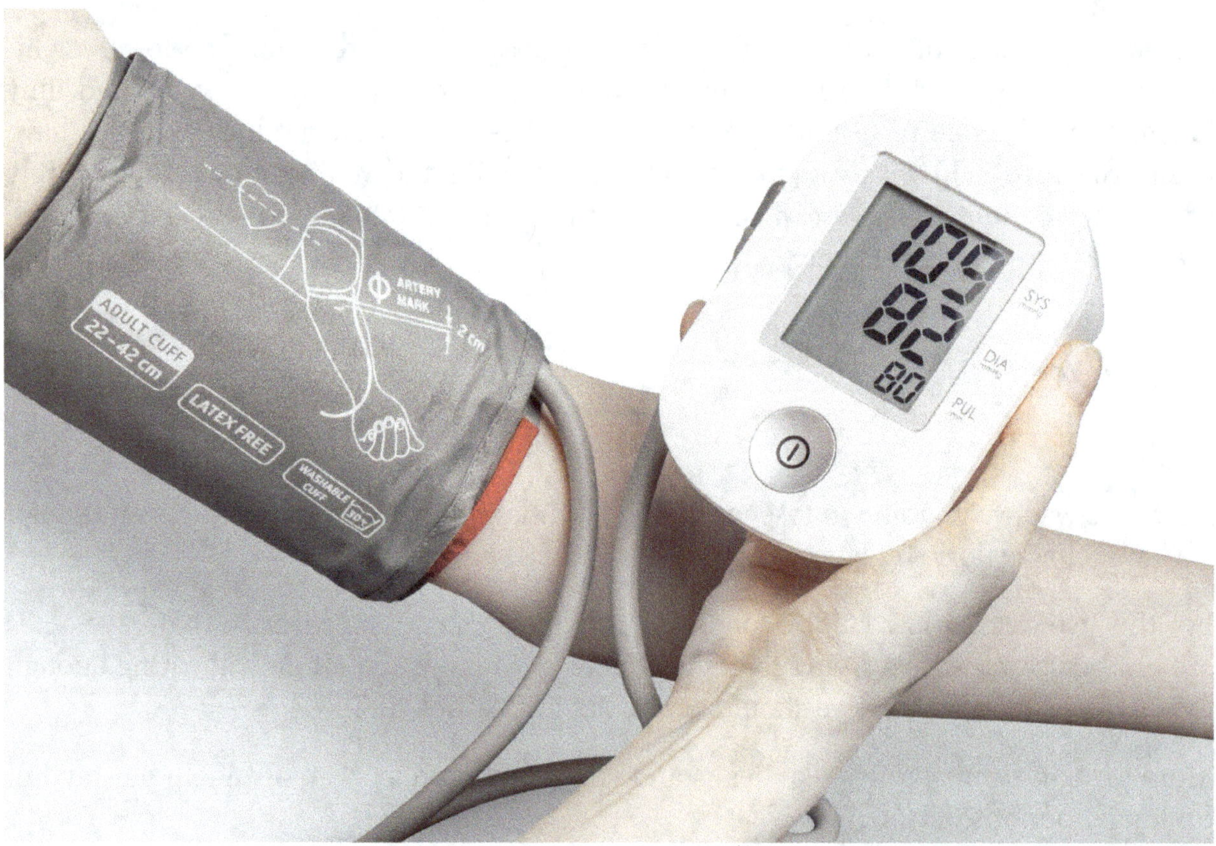

The first thing weight loss will do for you is lower your blood pressure. Being overweight or obese tends to naturally raise this, even if cholesterol and other levels are normal. Blood pressure can be a major risk factor for heart disease.

Reduces Heart Disease

Heart disease can pop up because of high cholesterol, high blood pressure, or simply because it's working too hard. All of these are factors that come with being overweight. Cholesterol, the fat deposits that cause blockages and clots within our arteries, reduces with weight loss (in addition to reducing because of the benefits that come with the Mediterranean diet). Blood pressure tends to be lower, as we mentioned above. Your heart may be working overtime to support your body if you are bigger too, which can tire it out.

Better Time in the Bedroom

Weight gain has been associated with erectile dysfunction and reduced orgasms, making sex not as enjoyable for all who wish to participate. By losing weight, you will see these things improve. This is a great example of where losing weight is just for yourself and not another person.

Mobility Increases

Another benefit of weight loss is that your ability to move improves. This does mean walking around and being able to run longer distances. This also means dancing becomes easier and more fun for you, and you're a better twister opponent. Being able to be more mobile can also help with things like balance and reducing clumsiness (unless, like me, you're naturally gifted in that area).

Improvements With Diabetes and Related Conditions

Type 2 diabetes has been tied to weight gain fairly often. Losing weight and dieting; however, can really help you with this. The diet itself and the resulting weight loss will lead to your blood sugar levels naturally dropping. Your body's ability to manage the food you are eating will naturally increase as well, especially if it isn't loaded with sugar.

This will help you if you are insulin resistant as well. It can help prevent type 2 diabetes from forming.

Lowered Cancer Risk

Some cancers, believe it or not, are thought to be brought on by obesity. Fat deposits get stuck in the lungs, liver, or other places that they shouldn't be. These settle and have the potential to mutate and grow into cancer. By losing weight, we reduce the chance of these fat deposits either gaining in strength and size or forming altogether.

Increased Energy

When we are overweight, we are literally carrying more weight with us throughout the day. Moving our body takes more energy. Thinking takes more energy. Doing daily tasks, you get the idea. By reducing our weight we are reducing the things we're carrying with us. As a result, we end up with more energy that we can spend doing various other things in our life.

Hormone Involvement

In previous sections we talked about the effect that food can have on our hormones, and how it makes certain processes within the body upset. Similar effects happen when we are overweight. Our body might start to make too much of one hormone and not enough of another. It might get mixed up on where certain hormones are supposed to go, and more. Generally, this causes us to be in even worse shape. When we start eating right and losing weight, our hormones tend to right themselves.

Improvements With Headaches and Migraines

Headaches and migraines are often caused by some of these hormone imbalances that we discussed in the previous section. If you get either headaches or migraines chronically, then it might be because of a hormone imbalance. Luckily, with weight loss, you are likely to see a major improvement in your symptoms.

Mood Booster

Guess what might affect our food? If your immediate thought at this point was "hormones" you're absolutely correct. Sadly, when our hormones are out of balance it negatively affects our mood in a negative way. Not only will weight loss help with the hormones, but the natural balance of eating right and exercising on their own has also proven to be a great mood booster.

Immune System

Our immune system's ability to function is based in part on our overall health. Simply put, if we aren't in good shape then neither is our immune system. If we are obese, then our immune system's ability to function is diminished. Hormones play a role in this as well. Weight Loss can help with these things. Eating right and exercising will play a big role in this too!

Skin

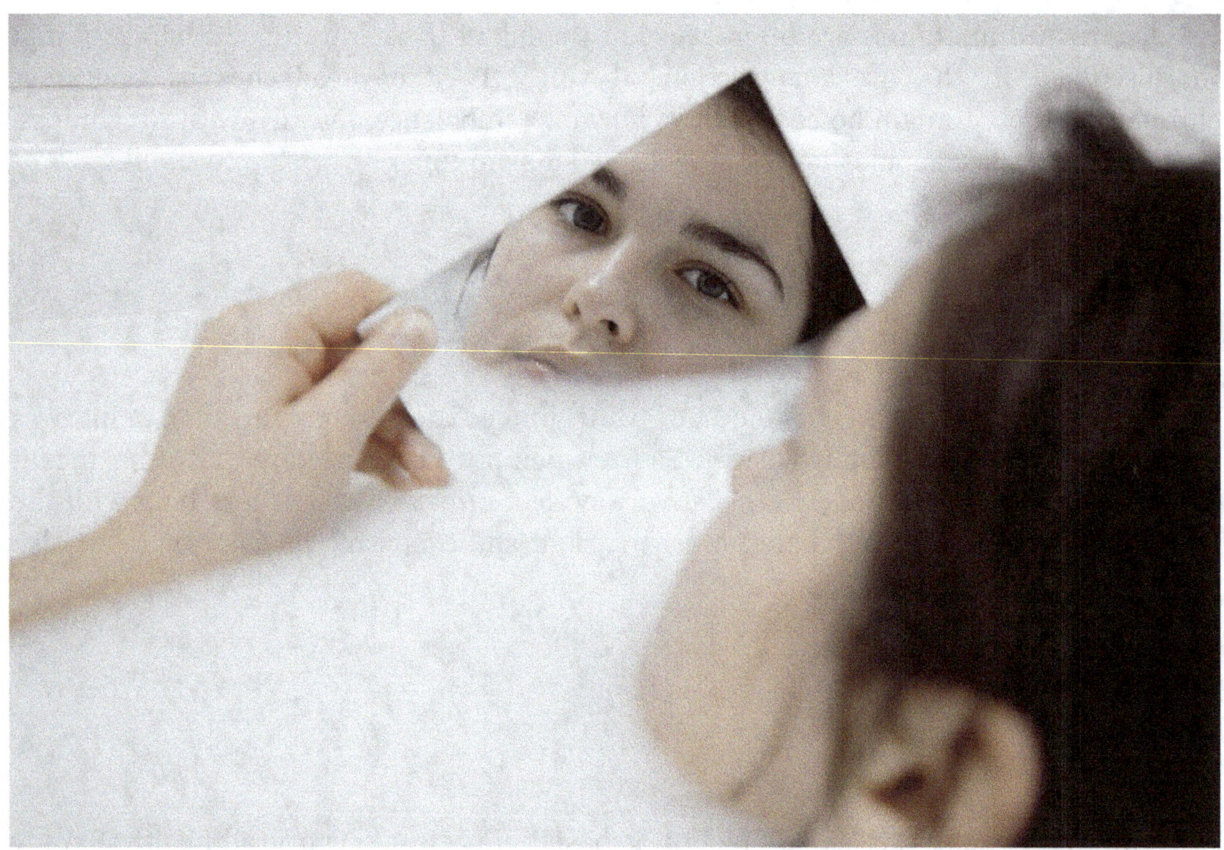

It probably comes as no surprise that our skin is a reflection of our hormones. If our hormones are imbalanced, our skin will show it in the form of acne. Luckily, this is an easy problem to fix with diet and weight loss. Not only will weight loss help the issue, but your diet will contain foods that are more beneficial for your skin.

Sleep

Sleep is affected by various things. In previous sections, we talked about both the effects of food and the effects of hormones on sleep. Both of these issues are eased when diet and weight loss come into play. Exercising for weight loss can also make you more tired throughout the day, leading you to sleep better.

Brain Function

We talked before about the toxic hormones and chemicals taking up residence in our brain. Being overweight, which causes your body to have even more hormonal issues—make this problem even worse. Losing weight can further help our body and brain get rid of these toxic things, and having a healthy diet can ensure that they are replaced with the right material for brain development.

Chronic Pain

Weight gain can actually be the cause of some chronic pain issues. We are putting more work on our bodies and causing pain from the strain it's going under. It's worth noting that hormones can also cause chronic pain, leading to some of your symptoms. Losing weight can help with both causes.

Appetite

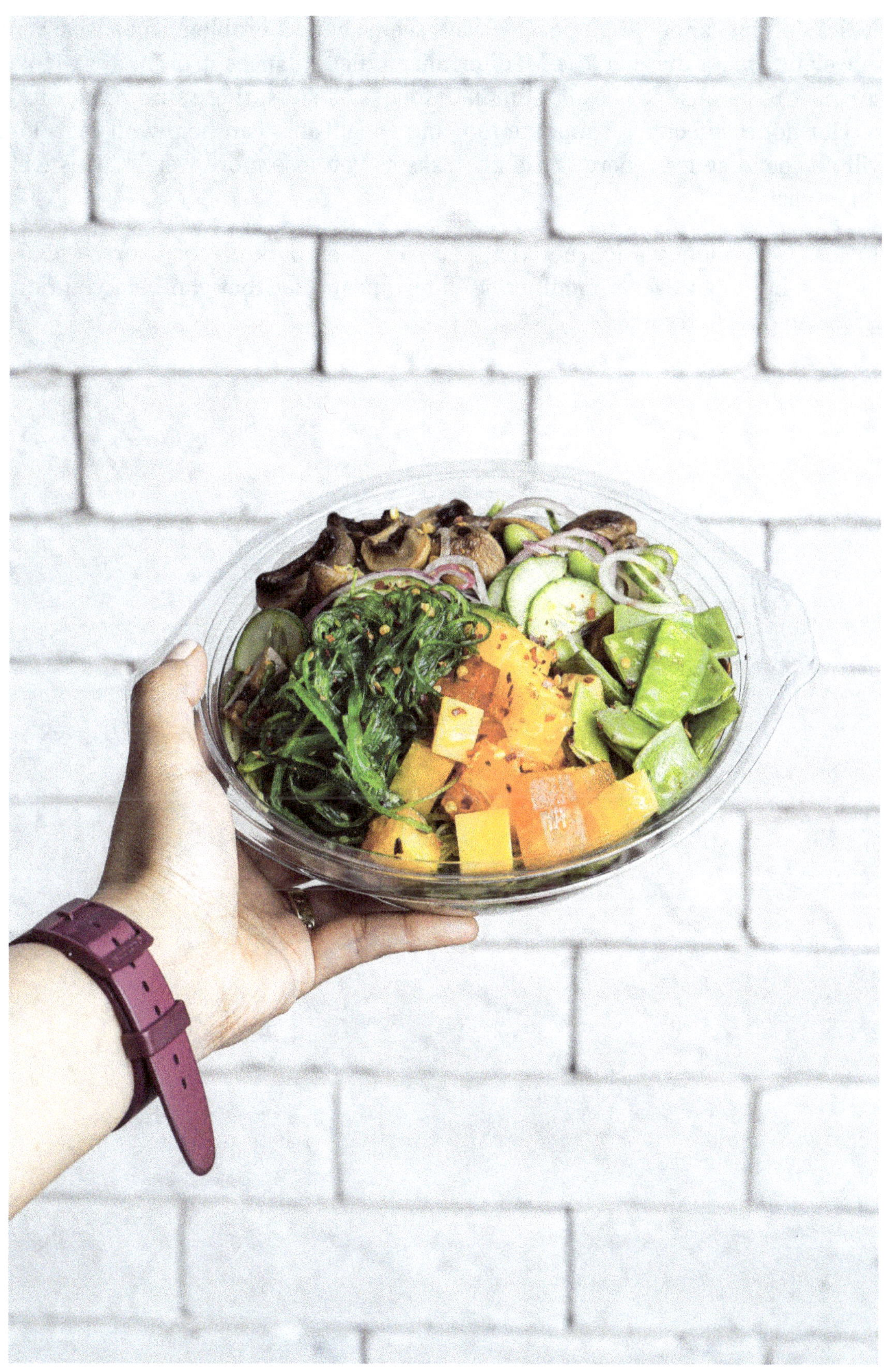

Finally, let's discuss appetite. Appetite always seems to be a problem when we are trying to lose weight. But, a diet like the Mediterranean diet balances itself in a way that will reduce appetite because it doesn't eliminate foods. As such, there's no reason to crave things. Hormones affect your appetite too, and weight loss can help with that. Finally, you will be spending less energy on daily tasks as you lose more weight. This will also have an impact.

Weight loss is absolutely a journey that you should embark on for yourself. Our next chapter is going to go over a modified Mediterranean diet that can help you out even more if you choose to try it!

Chapter 7: The Green Mediterranean Diet

One thing that I've mentioned before is that the Mediterranean diet is not automatically geared toward weight loss. The green Mediterranean diet makes a few key changes that make it much more weight-loss-friendly.

With the green Mediterranean diet, you are purposefully cutting out processed products, not just avoiding them. You are cutting out sweets entirely, including the pastries that might be found in these regions of the world. The placements of many things on the Mediterranean diet food pyramid changed. Let's take a look.

The Green Food Pyramid

Bottom Tier: Everyday foods

This bottom row is going to have a few similar ingredients on it.

First, of course, are vegetables. Vegetables are the cornerstone of many diets, and it likely comes as no surprise that you're going to have them even more often now.

Next, of course, are fruits. Again, both vegetables and fruits have a healthy dose of vitamins and minerals, and they should be included in your diet every single day.

In fact, it is recommended that either or both are added into every meal whenever possible. This means that you are eating them multiple times throughout the day.

Tier Two: Once a Day Foods

These foods should be a part of your diet really no more than once a day. The goal is to reduce fat and sugary carb consumption.

First up is whole grains. Making these a part of your diet once a day is fine and even encouraged since it has several needed vitamins and minerals, but if we add too many carbs to our diet, we are more likely to gain weight.

Nuts and seeds are on here too. Like whole grains, they contain nutrients that we need, but they can be high in carb or fat content. They tend to be a little over-processed in some parts of the world as well.

Finally, in the once-a-day category is olive oil. Olive oil has its benefits, but it is fat that can add to your waist. Using it to cook for just one meal can give the benefits without the consequences of having too much.

Tier Three: About Three Times a Week

What foods now come at the "three times a week" tier?

First off is fish. The placement of fish doesn't really change much here as it still has a lot of benefits.

Next up is legumes. These guys do provide some great protein, but some can be high in fat which is something that is important to watch for when we try to lose weight.

Our next item is red wine. Red wine in moderation is recommended in the traditional Mediterranean diet, and it simply suggests about a glass a day. The green Mediterranean diet goes a step further and limits it to about two to three times a week.

Tier Four: One to Two Times a Week

The position of poultry (white meat) hasn't really changed much either. Try to aim for two times a week at most.

Next up is dairy. This one is slightly more limited because dairy does tend to have a high fat content.

Rounding up this part of the party is eggs. Eggs move a little bit as well to just be consumed twice a week. In America, they are more processed, which is why their position changes.

Finally, on this list is red meat. Really, red meat in non-processed forms should really only be eaten once a week, thanks to its high fat content.

This last tier includes foods to essentially eliminate from your diet as they don't provide any benefits, but a host of issues come with them.

Sweets are on this list, sadly, but unsurprisingly.

Next on the list is anything processed. This includes processing done with refined grains or sugars, anything with added sugar, and processed meat such as lunch meat, spam, ground meat, sausages, and more (if you can't go out and cut it yourself, don't get it).

All of these are allowed in moderation in the traditional Mediterranean diet because it's culturally based. Its goal isn't to lose weight. But, when we are trying to lose weight, it's best to cut these items out.

The Wins of This Diet

Where does the green diet compare to the standard diet? Well, for you there will be a significant increase in fruit and vegetable intake. This can be a major benefit to your health. Both are low in calories, so you can eat a lot of them and fill yourself with satisfaction without having to deal with overspending calories. Now, second of all, you can get a lot more vitamins and minerals from your diet that you couldn't previously get.

Now, let's talk about your overall health. There is new research just starting to come out about animal foods, noting that there does seem to be a trend between animal foods and poor human health. This research is in its early stages, but many doctors are already suggesting that we try to limit animal foods as much as possible in order to see improvements in our overall health. The green diet goes a lot further to do this.

Now, in addition to our health, we are also helping our environment. Green seems to take on multiple meanings here, as research is also showing that the livestock industry is a significant contributor to pollution. Just the act of killing the animal will release carbon emissions into the air, and that doesn't get into the rest of the process that takes meat from the animal and puts it on our plate.

By reducing how much of it we eat, we reduce our overall carbon footprint. Today, actions like this are more important than ever!

Benefits

Some of the benefits that you get with the Mediterranean diet become even more pronounced with this diet!

Weight Loss

One of the great things about his diet is that it's geared even more toward weight loss than other diets are. By following this pattern, you will lose weight faster, and you are likely to see improvements in your overall metabolism. Since you are fighting fat, your gut size and health will improve too!

Heart Disease Risk

Your risk for heart disease will absolutely go down with this diet. This diet will cut down on animal products which have repeatedly been shown to have high fat contents that affect your blood pressure and cholesterol and lead to heart disease. With this diet, you will cut on those risk factors, which means that you are less likely to have a heart attack or develop other issues in the long run.

Diabetes

The Mediterranean diet already does some work with diabetes, and the restructuring of this diet makes these effects even more pronounced.

Inflammation

Inflammation and swelling can have a lot to do with our diet, especially when we eat a lot of processed, oily foods. The Green diet eliminates processed items, allowing for inflammation to decrease. This means less chronic pain and a healthier body for you.

Liver Health

Being overweight can really do a number on our liver! It increases fat deposits within it, which can lead to cancer, and everytime it can lead to liver failure. Not only does this diet help with weight loss, but it also focuses on foods that will actually help the liver to function better in the long run.

Alzheimer's and Dementia

Diet, obesity, and diabetes are all considered risk factors for Alzhiemer's and dementia. This diet works to fix all three, which can significantly reduce your risk. Now, if you have already been diagnosed, this diet can at least help slow the progression of it.

If you are really interested in weight loss, and you really want to see your health improve, I highly recommend you give this modified diet a try. Stick to other elements of the Mediterranean lifestyle, like exercise and family time, and you will definitely see a difference.

Conclusion

Our health is the most important thing in our life. Think about it. If we aren't healthy, then things aren't going to get done. We need our bodies to work for the rest of our life. For many of us, this means that we need to make some changes to the way we think about food and our lifestyle.

The Mediterranean diet has been one of my favorite diets to follow, and the main reason for this is that it isn't a diet at all. It was created by a random person online who wanted to make money. It was discovered by scientists who were just looking for the truth.

This diet focuses on fruits, vegetables, fish, olive oil, and freshness. It restructures food in a way that many diets don't, and this structure produces amazing benefits.

It isn't just the way they consume food that leads to more health within the Mediterranean region. It also has to do with their balance. They make time for exercise and family time, both of which have their own benefits.

It's thanks to this lifestyle that people have been able to see improvements in their heart conditions or they've been able to avoid one altogether.

People have been able to more successfully manage diabetes and reduce their risk of developing it. People have been able to better look after their overall organ health, especially in the case of their liver.

There is the fact that people are genuinely losing weight and keeping it off when they follow this eating pattern.

People are also experiencing mental and emotional benefits. Improved mood and mental health seem to come with this diet. The ability to better focus as we go through our work day can be seen as well. Our memory improves, and we end up with reduced risk for things like Alzheimer's and dementia.

Our body does better too. We can move more and do more and we process the food we take in better.

Don't all of these benefits sound amazing? Once you get into the swing of the Mediterranean diet, they can all be yours. All of the tools are here before you. All you need to do is get started.

References

35 Surprising Benefits of Weight Loss. (2017, November 15). Doctor Robert Marvin. https://doctormarvin.com/benefits-of-weight-loss/35-surprising-benefits-weight-loss/

Bjarnadottir, A. (2019, January 3). *9 Popular Weight Loss Diets Reviewed*. Healthline. https://www.healthline.com/nutrition/9-weight-loss-diets-reviewed#TOC_TITLE_HDR_6

CDC. (2019). *Healthy Eating for a Healthy Weight*. CDC. https://www.cdc.gov/healthyweight/healthy_eating/index.html

Centers for Disease Control and Prevention. (2021, September 27). Heart disease Facts. Centers for Disease Control and Prevention. https://www.cdc.gov/heartdisease/facts.htm

Contributor, L. A. (2021). To *"stay healthy and strong," a dietician eats these 5 staple foods of the Mediterranean diet*. CNBC. https://www.cnbc.com/2021/03/19/dietician-5-foods-of-the-mediterranean-diet-i-eat-to-stay-healthy-and-strong.html

Gunnars, K. (2021). *Mediterranean Diet 101: A Meal Plan and Beginner's Guide*. Healthline. https://www.healthline.com/nutrition/mediterranean-diet-meal-plan#bottom-line

Johnson, J. (2022, January 3). *Mediterranean diet: A guide and 7-day meal plan*. Www.medicalnewstoday.com. https://www.medicalnewstoday.com/articles/324221

Kingsland, J. (2022, March 22). *The green Mediterranean diet may protect health and the environment*. Www.medicalnewstoday.com. https://www.medicalnewstoday.com/articles/green-mediterranean-diet-could-be-a-win-win-for-health-and-the-planet

Migala, J. (2019, January 3). *What Is the Mediterranean Diet? Food List, Meal Plan, Benefits, More | Everyday Health*. EverydayHealth.com. https://www.everydayhealth.com/mediterranean-diet/guide/

Migala, J. (2021, March 9). *What Is the Green Mediterranean Diet, and Should You Try It?* Everyday Health. https://www.everydayhealth.com/mediterranean-diet/what-is-the-green-mediterranean-diet-and-should-you-try-it/

Nemati, Z. (2017). *Oh, may your silhouette never dissolve on the beach; may your eyelids never flutter into the empty distance. Don't leave me for a second, my dearest. Pablo Neruda.* In Unsplash. https://unsplash.com/photos/6sNQftdA3Zs

published, A. G. (2022, April 19). *How to follow a Mediterranean diet for weight loss.* Livescience.com. https://www.livescience.com/Mediterranean-diet-for-weight-loss

Seaver, D. V., M.S., & RD. (2022). *What Is a Green Mediterranean Diet—and Is It Healthy?* EatingWell. https://www.eatingwell.com/article/7957780/what-is-a-green-mediterranean-diet-and-is-it-healthy/

Secret benefits of weight loss. (n.d.). Www.piedmont.org. https://www.piedmont.org/living-better/secret-benefits-of-weight-loss

Shubhangi. (2021, March 9). *Weight Loss Diet: 10 Best Different Types of Diet to Lose Weight.* Wellcurve Blog. https://www.wellcurve.in/blog/best-weight-loss-diet-to-get-in-shape/?gclid=CjwKCAjwoMSWBhAdEiwAVJ2ndkwUSpWXd7pCrG-TWFKaQZGNajGogVYxhinDSg9FGix--Pr9il3O2xoCb7UQAvD_BwE

Image References

Aceron, E.-S. (2020). *Poke Bowl.* In Unsplash. https://unsplash.com/photos/NnIWIPdxbPg

Akyurt, E. (2021). *delicious traditional veggie pastas on plate.* In Unsplash. https://unsplash.com/photos/X4QCAodTlho

Barcelo, C. (2019). *A woman doing a yoga pose.* In Unsplash. https://unsplash.com/photos/nqUHQkuVj3c

Diabetesmagazijn.nl. (2020). *Complete set for glucose measurement (diabetes). Glucometer, lancing device, strips and lancets.* In Unsplash. https://unsplash.com/photos/z03Q6GAkqKM

Grabkowska, M. (2017). *carrot cake smoothie.* In Unsplash. https://unsplash.com/photos/qobKY_4FANw

Hieb, A. (2016). *Overnight Oats.* In Unsplash. https://unsplash.com/photos/LzrMzmVWhJw

Leunen, S. (2020). *Girl in a mirror*. In unsplash. https://unsplash.com/photos/rXEY6McWiAs

Lewis, C. (2017). *Spices*. In Unspalsh. https://unsplash.com/photos/vA1L1jRTM70

Lim, A. (2021). *Fish Tacos*. In Unsplash. https://unsplash.com/photos/aUWCL1DtMtM

liu. (2020). *Rice dish*. In unsplash. https://unsplash.com/photos/tSw7MaGGJDs

Mockup graphics. (2020). *Clean medical tonometer with hands on white background*. In Unsplash. https://unsplash.com/photos/i1iqQRLULlg

nrd. (2018). Vegetable shelf. In Unsplash. https://unsplash.com/photos/D6Tu_L3chLE

Olsson, E. (2018a). Easy Chocolate Oatmeal Breakfast. In Unsplash. https://unsplash.com/photos/3_qr5tJOIbs

Olsson, E. (2018b). Made using all plant-based, wholesome ingredients. In Unsplash. https://unsplash.com/photos/_Buh5P_61JE

Podvalny, A. (2016). Various vegetables in Srilanka. In unsplash. https://unsplash.com/photos/WOxddhzhC1w

Primeau, N. (2018). Veggie Bowl. In Unsplash. https://unsplash.com/photos/-ftWfohtjNw

Ramos, S. (2020). *Body Weight Scale*. In Unsplash. https://unsplash.com/photos/mz9koyBQd4Q

Rendina, D. (2018). *Yogurt Bowl*. In Unspalsh. https://unsplash.com/photos/SH6vc3VOOwE

Tursunov, B. (2022). *Piece of salmon fish frying on hot pan with sizzling oil at home kitchen*. In Unsplash. https://unsplash.com/photos/1aj1sirGQAA